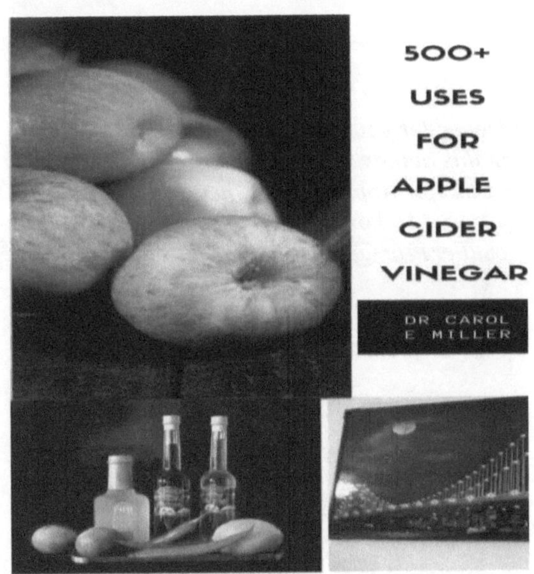

500+ USES FOR APPLE CIDER VINEGAR

DR CAROL E MILLER

APPLES USED AS PROVERBS

PROVERBS 25:11

[11]A WORD FITLY SPOKEN IS LIKE APPLES OF GOLD IN PICTURES OF SILVER.

SONG OF SOLOMON 2:5

[5]STAY ME WITH FLAGONS, COMFORT ME WITH APPLES: FOR I AM SICK OF LOVE.

SONG OF SOLOMON 7:8

[8]I SAID, I WILL GO UP TO THE PALM TREE, I WILL TAKE HOLD OF THE BOUGHS THEREOF: NOW ALSO

THY BREASTS SHALL BE AS CLUSTERS OF THE VINE, AND THE SMELL OF THY NOSE LIKE APPLES;

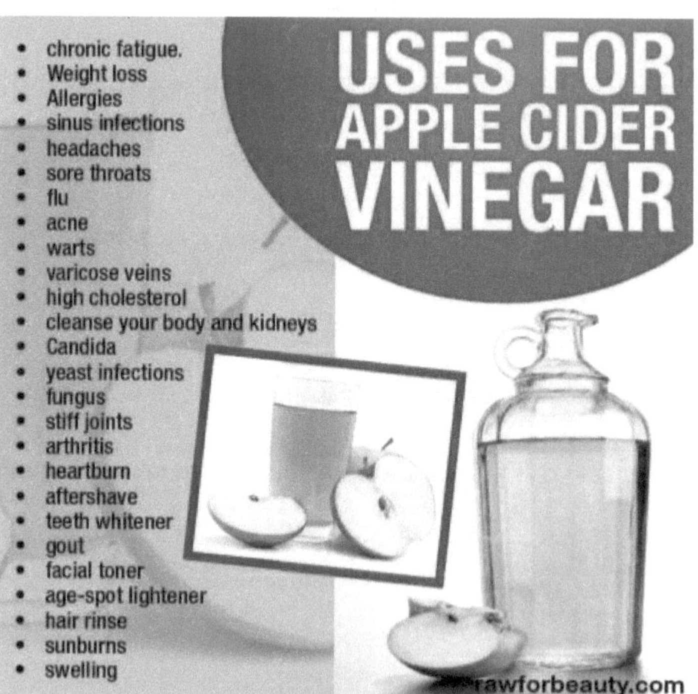
USES FOR
APPLE CIDER
VINEGAR
chronic fatigue.
Weight loss
Allergies
sinus infections
headaches
sore throats
flu
acne
warts
varicose veins
high cholesterol
cleanse your body and kidneys
Candida
yeast infections
fungus
stiff joints
arthritis
heartburn
aftershave
teeth whitener
gout
facial toner
age-spot lightener
hair rinse
sunburns
swelling
rawforbeauty.com

TABLE OF CONTENTS

Disclaimer: this book is NOT intended to be a comprehensive or

exhaustive analysis of apple cider vinegar.

Additionally, there are also downsides to

consuming too much vinegar.

The expression, "An apple a day keeps the doctor away," is applicable to the benefits of apple cider vinegar. An old European folk tale says, "An apple a day keeps the doctor begging for bread."

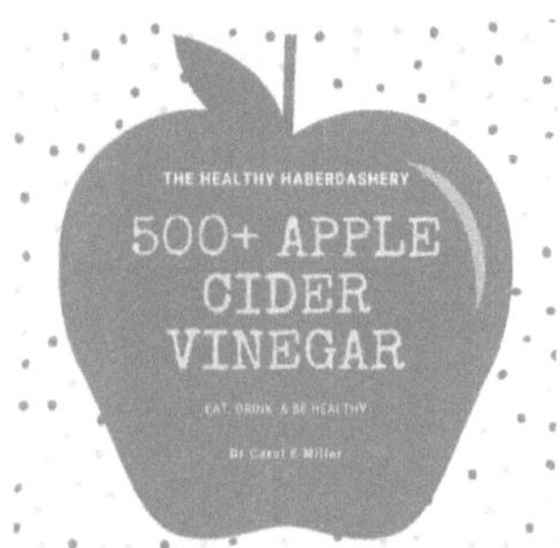

Apple Cider Vinegar (ACV), has proved to be one of the most important ingredients in my Detoxification regimen. *The word vinegar comes from the French vin aigre; it was actually called aceto, meaning "acid," by the Romans.* The history of apple cider is chronicled as far back as 1300 BC. Geologists and historians purport that apple trees adorned the Niles River Delta.

The Miraculous Superiority of Vinegar!

Folklore has it that there are magical powers using Vinegar? It can be uncanny! In fact, this product can battle as many problems as Vinegar. It is a gift from The Most High to cure most ailments for the detoxification of the overall health for our bodies.

The astronomical number of ailments that you can eliminate toxins and/or alleviate pain with this everyday product is truly a blessing. And the fact that it is still so cheap it's truly unbelievable for it multifunctional properties! You can literally get rid of many costly domestic products once you've discovered the magical powers of apple cider vinegar and its descendant, white distilled vinegar.

Cure Your Ailments the Natural Way

Since Vinegar is such a natural product, you can really benefit from its impact without the side effects of chemical compounds. Please read about the wonderful benefits! It is one of the ingredients that is part of many products today. Make it a part of your overall health regime!

APPLE CIDER VINEGAR (ACV)	
MINERALS & TRACE ELEMENTS:	
Calcium	Chlorine
Copper	Fluorine
Iron	Potassium
Magnesium	Phosphorus
Sodium	Vitamins A
Vitamins B1	Vitamins B2
Vitamins B6	Vitamins C
Vitamins F	Vitamins E

TRACE MINERALS

The Trace elements Are bio elements or micronutrients (small amounts) present in all living beings,

being chemical elements that are necessary in almost any living particle to function properly.

BENEFITS OF VITAMINS & MINERALS

PAUL BRAGG, N.D. PHD described ACV to promote youthful skin & a vibrant body.

Helps remove artery plaque & eliminates toxin & fights germs, bacteria, virus & mold naturally.

Helps regulate calcium deposits & metabolism to promote good digestion & Ph balance.

THIS BOOK PROMOTES THE FIGHTING OF ARTHRITIS, ACHES AND PAINS.

BENEFITS OF VITAMINS & MINERALS

No matter the age, but specifically the well-aged, our bodies require vital minerals and vitamins for

every process and function. These nutrients work in together to grow, heal, repair and maintain your

body's cells, organs, systems and skeleton. Therefore, they interact to promote good health and

wellness as they are responsible for maintaining, or assisting with, the proper functionality of many of

the various bodily functions that are required to sustain life.

APPLE CIDER VINEGAR & WEIGHT LOSS

APPLE CIDER IS THE NAME USED IN THE US AND CANADA

FOR AN UNFILTERED, UNSWEETENED,

NON-ALCOHOLIC BEVERAGE MADE FROM APPLES.

Those who consumed 1 tablespoon (15 ml) of vinegar per day had on average the following benefits:

- **Weight loss:** 2.6 pounds (1.2 kg)

- **Decrease in body fat percentage:** 0.7%

- **Decrease in waist circumference:** 0.5 in (1.4 cm)

- **Decrease in triglycerides:** 26%

This is what changed in those consuming 2 tablespoons (30 ml) of vinegar per day:

- **Weight loss:** 3.7 pounds (1.7 kg)

- **Decrease in body fat percentage:** 0.9%

- **Decrease in waist circumference:** 0.75 in (1.9 cm)

- **Decrease in triglycerides:** 26%

Obese people who took

1–2 tablespoons (15–30 ml)

of apple cider vinegar

daily for 12 weeks lost weight and body fat on average.

Study of apple cider vinegar

<u>**APPLE CIDER VINEGAR & WEIGHT LOSS**</u>

Improve metabolic production

Reduce dangerous LDL cholesterol

Diminish water retention

Alleviate excessive sodium from the body

Reduce premature calcification of the arteries

Amplify energy and vitality

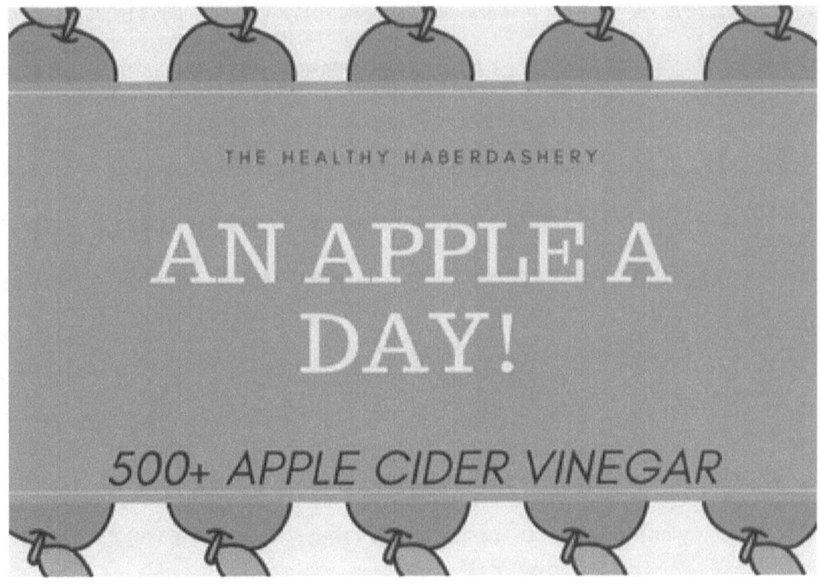

<u>A DELICIOUS BEVERAGE</u>

IN THE MIDST OF ITS DISCOVERY IN GREAT BRITAIN.

THE JUICE OF THE FRUIT WAS HEALTHFULNESS.

<u>MY ARTHRITIS COCKTAIL</u>

During the past couple of years, I have experienced a feeling of well-being and respite from pain! **MY ARTHRITIS COCKTAIL** will invigorate the body, thereby reducing aches and pains. It will improve blood circulation and aid in the Detoxification process. Although, it will not prevent conditions from re-occurring it is an excellent addition to your detoxification regimen.

Thank The Most High God for these NATURAL healing apples! MY ARTHRITIS COCKTAIL has enabled me to feel more energized. I have found the HOLY GRAIL OF THE FOUNTAIN OF YOUTH! I now have a FRESH LEASE ON LIFE. For all those that are still skeptical, YOU MUST NOT LOSE HOPE! Just make a gallon of the Arthritis Cocktail. Start drinking 1 glass and drink up to 3 glasses per day.

The brand that I have been using for over many years is Bragg Apple Cider Vinegar (with the mother). For years, it has been part of my **DETOXIFICATION PROGRAM**. I really believe that the discovery of this product helps to break down the deposits within my blood stream to keep my cholesterol under control.

DETOXIFICATION PROGRAM

Specific program designed to support energy metabolism (absorption) and enhance the body's natural metabolic detoxification process, which are scientifically-based method to help simplify the removal of undesirable toxins from the body.

10

MY ARTHRITIS COCKTAIL

MY ARTHRITIS COCKTAIL has enabled me to STRIDE BRISKLY instead of dawdling or plodding along! This wonderful product has eased my agonizing aches and pains. I have had 3 serious sciatic episodes, which caused me to be bedridden! I even began to use motorized carts when I shopped. I underwent surgery for torn ligaments in my knees, but still experienced major pain. I began to take a many anti-inflammatory drugs & then cortisone (ouch!) shot to no avail!

SCIATICA PAIN

Sciatica is a common type of pain affecting the sciatic nerve, a large nerve extending from the lower back down the back of each leg. This pain may go down the back, outside, or front of the leg. It feels like a long hot coal running from your thigh to your spine, it's horrible pain!

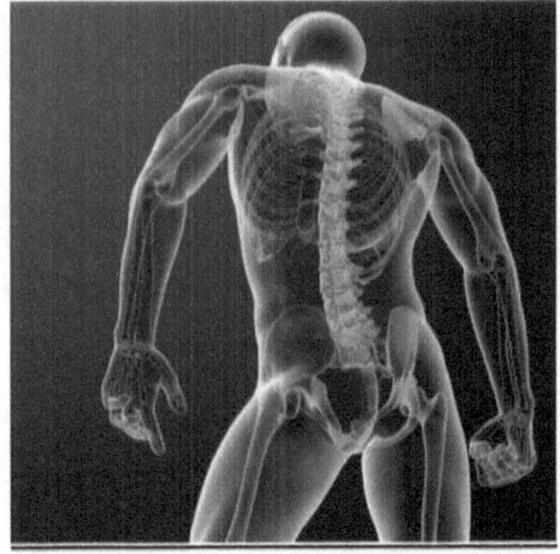

That's when I decided to go on my own quest and created this wonderful Detoxification drink! MY ARTHRITIS COCKTAIL is a purifier and is effective in promoting the health of organs such as the bladder, kidneys and liver by helping to prevent excessive alkaline in the urine.

(Do not take plain vinegar before breakfast or ingest white vinegar).

But you can take MY ARTHRITIS COCKTAIL anytime; especially when you're tired!

My customers, who utilized this

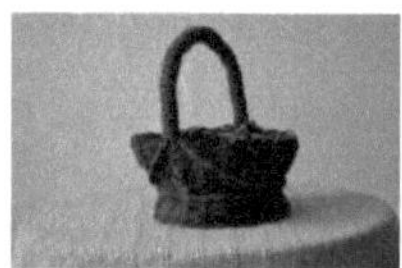

through my company,

The Healthy Haberdashery

were ecstatic.

I sold PAIN RELIEF BASKETS and my clients

encouraged me to make the

ACV (apple cider vinegar) information available &

I decided to take it Internationally!

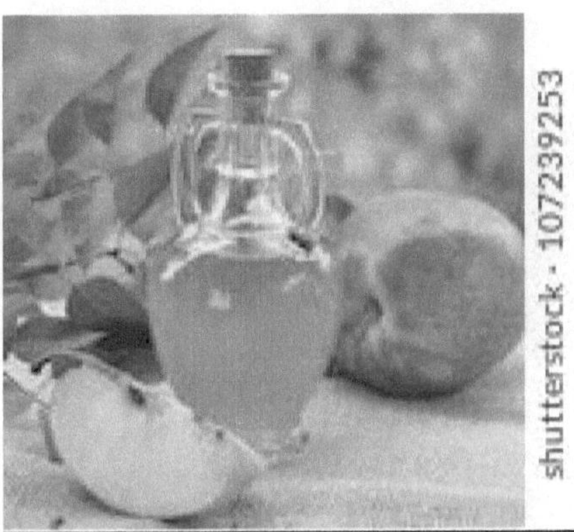

ONE THREE GLASSES (DAILY)

My Arthritis Cocktail #1

8 oz. Water – warm or glass

to mix the water & honey

1 to 2 teaspoons of Apple Cider Vinegar

1 to 2 teaspoons of Honey (Stevia).

Sweeten to Taste & Enjoy!

My Lazy Arthritis Vinegar #2

Elixir (Gallon=Weekly)

1 Gallon Pure Water

½ Cup of Apple Cider Vinegar

(Increase as desired)

16 Oz Honey:

Mix Raw Honey &

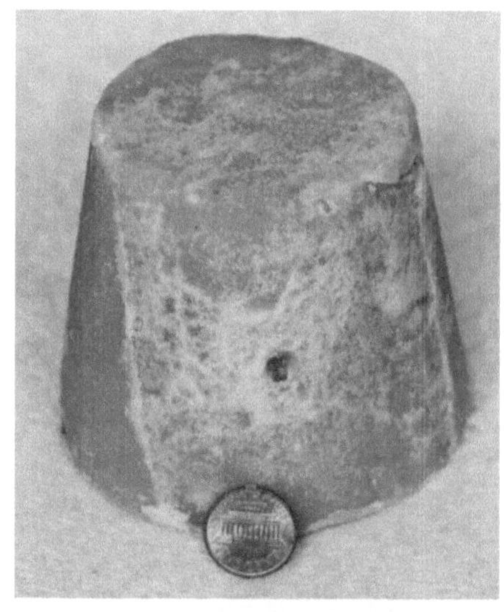

Apple Cider vinegar

First in a separate picture,

Then add this to water!)

<u>**My Super Lazy Arthritis Vinegar #3**</u>
<u>**Elixir (Gallon=Weekly)**</u>

½ Gallon Apple Cider Vinegar

(Raw & Unfiltered @ grocer)

Mix Raw Apple Cider vinegar

(Mix until you cannot taste

Apple Cider Vinegar, Voila!)

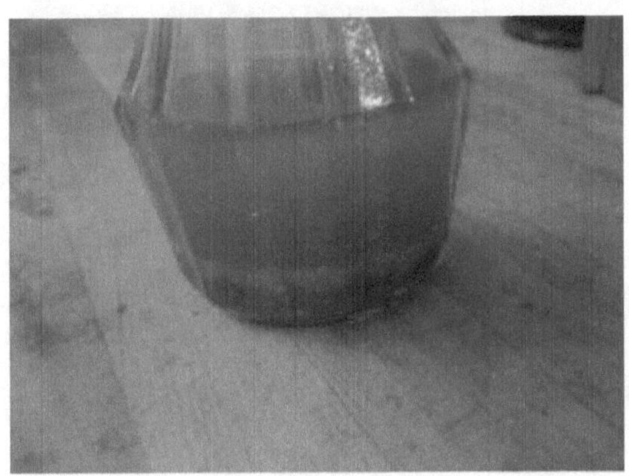

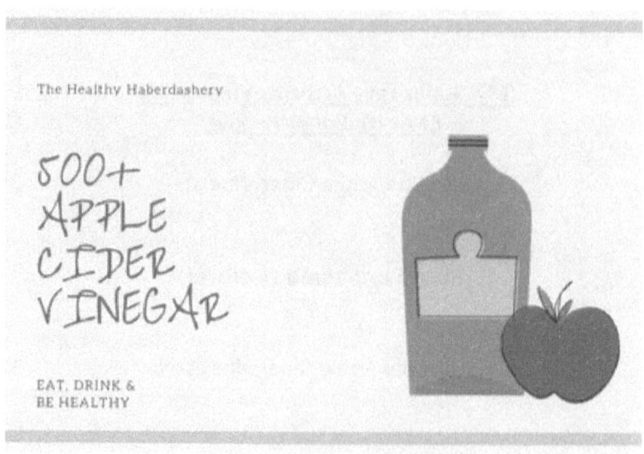

APPLE CIDER VINEGAR

Apple cider vinegar has been used in cooking

and natural medicine for thousands of years.

Many claim it has health benefits,

including **WEIGHT LOSS & PAIN**..

8 OUNCES OF APPLE CIDER VINEGAR:
98.9% water

34 calories

No fat

Trace of protein & pectin fiber

14.2 grams of carbohydrate

14 mg. calcium (less than 2% of USRDA)

22 mg. Phosphorus

1.4 mg. iron

2 mg. sodium

240 mg. potassium (half of what is in a banana)

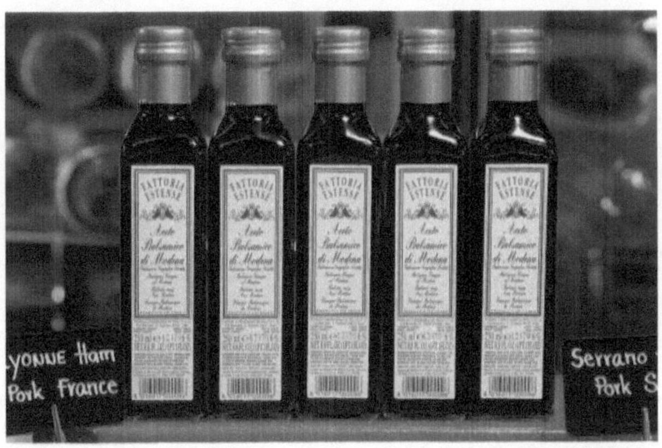

1. <u>Apple Cider:</u> made from apples with the MOTHER OF VINEGAR because of its health properties.

2. <u>Balsamic</u> – made from white grapes; an aged type of vinegar; casks are made various types of wood; oak, mulberry, chestnut cherry, juniper, ash, and acacia.

3. <u>Beer</u> – Vinegar made from beer is produced in Germany, Austria, the Netherlands and Bavaria.

4. <u>Cane</u> – made from sugar cane juice, contains no residual sugar; produced in France and USA.

5.<u>Coconut</u> – made from the sap of the coconut tree; used in the Asian culture in the Philippines.

6. <u>Date</u> – made from dates; a traditional product of the Middle East.

7. <u>East Asian Black</u> – Chinese black vinegar is an aged produce made from rice, wheat, millet or sorghum.
8. <u>Fruit Flavored vinegars</u> – infused with raspberries, blueberries, or figs, blood orange and pear.

9. <u>Fruit</u> –white grapes; casks are types of wood; oak, mulberry, chestnut, cherry juniper, ash and acacia.

10.<u>Honey</u> – commercially produced in Italy & France & all International Global Countries.

11.<u>Herb vinegars</u> – flavored with herbs, such as the   Mediterranean herbs of thyme and oregano.

12.<u>Kombucha</u> – Probiotic vinegar, culture of yeast & bacteria promote a healthy digestive tract.

KOMBUCHA HONEY

Kombucha as opposed to regular kombucha is because jun kombucha is made using green tea and honey rather than black tea and cane sugar. Green tea is well-known for its health benefits, and honey is a natural sugar with good-for-you nutrients.

13.<u>Malt</u> – made from malting barley, ale is brewed for liquor.

14.<u>Raisin</u> –raisins used in the cuisines of the Middle East; produced in the Middle East in Turkey.

15.<u>Rice:</u> from rice in sushi; white, light yellow, red & black variants for sushi rice & salad dressings.

16.<u>Sweetened vinegar</u> by the Cantonese is made from rice wine, sugar and herbs, ginger and cloves.

17.<u>Spiced vinegar</u> – produced in the Philippines is flavored with chili peppers, onions, and garlic.

18.<u>White</u> –grain (often maize) & water; this acetate in water is normally 5% acetic acid solution for culinary.

RED WINE

WHITE WINE;

CHAMPAGNE,

SHERRY,

PINOT

APPLE CIDER VINEGAR COCKTAIL

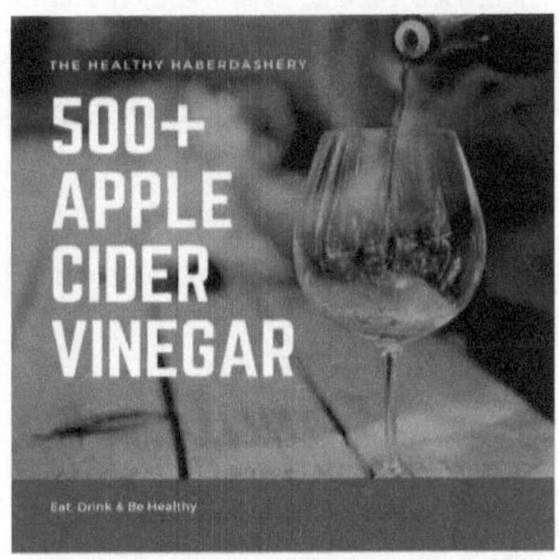

THEREARE 500+

GREAT BENEFITS OF

APPLE CIDER VINEGAR

There are many superior benefits from sipping apple cider vinegar (ACV)! Without a doubt, it's one of the most amazing benefits is that it is thought to regulate blood sugar levels, improve weight loss, more importantly, it reduces the any additional weight gain.

Significantly, there is an improvement in stomach ailments for gut health. The lowering of cholesterol levels has been noted, and the enhancement of facial PH levels in the skin health. Apple Cider Vinegar is a type of vinegar made from ripe, freshly crushed, apples.

Apple cider vinegar (ACV) has become the go(buy in grocery stores, health food stores) -to (homeopathic cure-all for a range of medical ailments, such as indigestion and yeast infections.

Homeopathy or homeopathy is a pseudoscientific classification of alternative medicine. It was created in 1796 by Samuel Hahnemann. Its practitioners, called homeopaths, believe that a substance that causes symptoms of a disease in healthy people would cure similar symptoms in sick people.

Below is a YouTube videos on how to make Homemade vinegar.

HOW TO MAKE

APPLE CIDER VINEGAR

MADE IN YOUR HOME

HOMEMADE APPLE CIDER

VINEGAR REAL RECIPE (ACV)

PLEASE REVIEW YOUTUBE

PLEASE COPY AND PASTE TO VIEW VIDEO:

https://youtu.be/WM9J5cxKkas

<u>**ANCIENTS BENEFITED FROM VINEGAR**</u>

Vinegar is one of nature's great gifts to mankind, and vinegar history shows us why. It is a truly natural product. Any alcoholic beverage, whether it is made from apples, grapes, dates, rice or plain white sugar, once exposed to air, will **turn naturally** to **vinegar.** It is the ever-present bacteria in the air that converts the alcohol in cider, wine, and beer, into **acetic acid** , lactic acid and propionic acid promote digestion, balance acid/alkaline levels of the blood, detoxify the body, dissolve fats, kills viruses, bacteria and fungus.

3).In the midst of its alleged discovery in **Great Britain**, the juice of the fruit was a CURIOUS BEVERAGE.

4). Ancient documents detail that when the **Romans traveled to England**, they observed the Kentish villagers enjoying the delicious CIDER JUICE.

5). The industry of cider apple production was widespread in **Great Britain after the Norman** Conquest (1066). Apple Cider Vinegar was used in the ancient civilization of Egypt, Babylonia and the Roman Empire, it was used for every medical condition from simple DIGESTIVE PROBLEMS to EXTERNAL WOUND CARE.

6). As the acidity of the compound is a bit harsh to consume, the advantages of apple cider vinegar can be enjoyed in many weight loss products like **THERMADROL.**

7). Recorded vinegar history starts around **5000 BC, when the Babylonians** were using the fruit of the date palm to make WINE AND VINEGAR.

8). They used it as a AS A PRESERVING OR PICKLING AGENT. Vinegar residues have been found in ancient **Egyptian urns traced to 3000 BC**. Recorded vinegar history in China starts from texts dated back to 1200 BC.

9). During **BIBLICAL TIMES**, vinegar was used to FLAVOR FOODS, as an energizing drink, and as a medicine, and it is mentioned in both the old and new testaments. For example, after working hard gleaning barley in the fields, Ruth was invited by Boaz to eat bread and dip it in vinegar. (Ruth 2:14)

<u>**ANCIENTS BENEFITED FROM VINEGAR: HIPPOCRATES, CHRISTOPHER COLUMBUS**</u>

<u>HIPPOCRATES AND ACV</u>

Hippocrates used vinegar to treat 17 different conditions, ranging from ulcers to fractures

10).   **In ancient Greece**, around 400 BC, Hippocrates, the father of modern medicine, prescribed apple cider vinegar mixed with honey for a **variety of ills**, including coughs and colds.

<u>CHRISTOPHER COLUMBUS AND ACV</u>

It's recorded Christopher Columbus carried it in barrels on his voyages

11).   Christopher Columbus and crew on his first voyage to discover America in 1492 had vinegar barrels for Scurvy.

12). **The ancients** were quick to explore the remarkable versatility of vinegar. In 5,000 B.C. the Babylonians were fermenting the fruit of date palms to make date vinegar and used it as a preservative.

13). The **Ancient Egyptians** sang the praises of vinegar as far back as 3,000 B.C. One Egyptian jar dating back to 8,000 B.C.

14).   Records show that the **Egyptians were using ACV** not just as an antiseptic, but as a weight loss as well.

<u>**CLEOPATRA AND APPLE CIDER VINEGAR**</u>

Apple Cider Vinegar: Cleopatra used apple cider vinegar to promote blood circulation and maintains the pH of the skin. Therefore, she used Apple Cider Vinegar for face rinsing.

15). In later times, Cleopatra demonstrated vinegar's solvent property by dissolving precious pearls in it to win a wager that she could consume a fortune in a single meal.

16). **In ancient Greece,** Hippocrates strongly advocated drinking vinegar for his patients as an energizing tonic and a healing elixir.

17). *OXYMEL,* a medicine he often prescribed, was a combination of honey and vinegar; he instructed his students that they would find the drink very useful for expelling phlegm and promoting freedom of breathing.

18). **Caesar's armies** used sweetened, diluted vinegar called *posca* (poor man's wine) as a preventative medicine (much as we take vitamins today) and to cook with.

19). They used it for its antiseptic properties against insect & snakebites and to clean their wounds after battle (a life-saving practice emulated as recently as **World War I**).

20). In the **second century A.D.**, Galen prescribed the combination of honey and vinegar for coughs.

21). During the **Sung dynasty** in ancient China, vinegar was listed by Tzu-Mu as one of the seven necessities that even the poorest people couldn't do without.

22). **Ancient Japanese** documentation has vinegar reaching an art form in the Heian Period with the addition of vinegar from fruits and flowers.

23). In **Paris by the middle ages,** it was sold by street vendors as a body deodorant and healing tonic.

24). In the **17th century, Europeans** discovered the medicinal value of vinegar and prepared antiseptic vinegar, vinegar syrups and a variety of medical types of vinegar.

25). In 1703, B. Boyles, a fellow of the Royal Society of London, recommended vinegar as a gargle.
(ACV) BENEFITS FOR THE MILITARY

Vinegar history provides many examples of this liquid's usefulness to soldiers

such as an **energizing tonic** used throughout the ages.

26). It is also recorded that Hannibal used vinegar to remove boulders in his path while crossing the Alps by heating the boulders & pouring cold vinegar which cracked them into stones.

28). Roman soldiers called this refreshing drink **"posca"**, and used it regularly as did the Japanese samurai. The addition of vinegar to drinking water had the additional benefit of killing any **infectious agents** that might have been present.

29). Throughout history the **antiseptic nature** of vinegar has been used to clean and disinfect soldiers to speed up **healing.**

30). Vinegar's **dissolving power** was use by the Carthaginian Hannibal when to dissolve snow and ice.

31). **LOUIS XIII OF FRANCE** (1601-1643) is reported to have paid 1.3 million francs for the vinegar used to cool the military cannons.

32).During the middle ages, vinegar along with an abrasive material such as sand; was used to clean flexible mail armor.

33). VINEGAR & THE BUBONIC PLAGUE

From 1347 to 1771 many European cities were repeatedly hit by the bubonic plague. It is estimated that about 50 million people died in all from this disease which spread from rats to man by infected fleas.

In 1721, the Bubonic Plague hit many French cities so hard that all the dead could not be decently buried. To cope with this situation, the French authorities released convicts from prison to help bury infectious corpses.

According to legend, while most died, one team of four convicted thieves managed to survive by drinking daily large amounts of vinegar infused with garlic. As a result, vinegar steeped in garlic is still sold today as **four thieves' vinegar.**

34). By holding vinegar-soaked sponges to their noses, European aristocrats of the seventeenth and eighteenth centuries were able to ward off the noxious odors of outdoor garbage and raw sewage.

35). Small silver boxes called vinaigrettes were used to carry these sponges and they were also stored in special compartments in the heads of walking canes.

36). Around 40 BC legend has it that Cleopatra, queen of Egypt, won a wager with the roman general Mark Anthony, when after a lavish meal, she dissolved a priceless pearl in vinegar and then drank the resulting solution. By doing this she proved that she could provide a feast for the two of them that would cost a fortune

APPLE CIDER VINEGAR SIGNIFICANCE

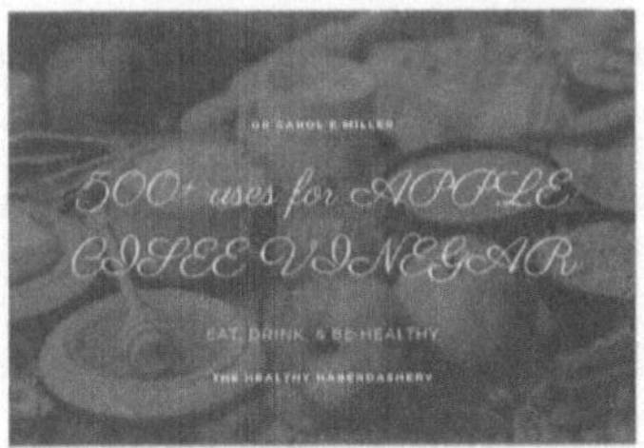

There are historical records showing a myriad of uses for apple cider vinegar from

All over the world (rose, 2006). balancing the skin's PH apple cider vinegar also has a

Long history of cosmetic use and it was frequently found in beauty products throughout the ages,

Starting in roman times when it was said to be used as a toner.

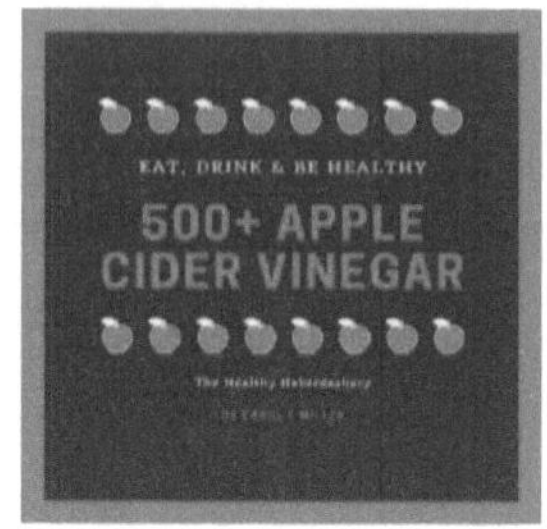

AN APPLE A DAY SYNDROME!
USES FOR APPLE CIDER VINEGAR

Apple cider (also called sweet cider or soft cider or simply cider) is the name used in the United States and parts of Canada for an unfiltered, unsweetened, non-alcoholic beverage made from apples. Though typically referred to simply as "cider" in those areas, it is not to be confused with the alcoholic beverage known as cider in other places, which is "hard cider" in the US and Canada

AN APPLE A DAY SYNDROME

It turns out that eating an apple a day really does keep the doctor away -- but you've got to eat the peel. And no fair skipping the apple altogether in favor of a megadose of more health benefits from eating whole fruits. When experiencing antioxidant activity, you get a variety of antioxidants. Antioxidants are substances that can prevent or slow damage to cells to combat toxicity."

<u>VINEGAR GOES COMMERCIAL BIG TIME!</u>

37). In 1394, a group of French vintners developed a continuous method for making vinegar called the **Orleans method.** Oak barrels were used as fermentation vessels and the vinegar was siphoned off through a spigot at the bottom of the barrel.

38). The New Orleans method left about 15% of the vinegar which contained the " concentrated bacteria floating on top A new batch of cider or wine was carefully added to the barrel and was quickly started by the remaining vinegar.

39). The French vintners formed a guild of master vinegar makers, using this Orleans method, they were better able to supply vinegar market.

40).The vinegar industry in Europe flourished during the renaissance and many flavored vinegars were made with various **spices, herbs, fruits** and **even flowers**. By the eighteenth century there were over one hundred varieties of **infused vinegars** available.

41). Vinegar was well known to the European alchemists of the middle ages. By pouring it over lead, they made a sweet tasting substance they called **"sugar of lead"**, which was used well into the nineteenth century to smooth and sweeten a harsh cider.

<u>SUGAR OF LEAD POURED OVER APPLE CIDER VINEGAR</u>

Centuries ago in Europe, the sugar of lead sweetener agent was used for wine (remember, they didn't have boxes of granulated sugar in those days) by pouring vinegar over lead, which was called "sugar of lead." It of course was highly poisonous. a story worth remembering about the importance of using vinegar judiciously.

42). Several varieties of **wild crab apple** are native to North America, but it was the western European settlers who introduced the larger, more useful **dessert** and **cider apples.**

WILLIAM BLACKSTONE AND APPLES

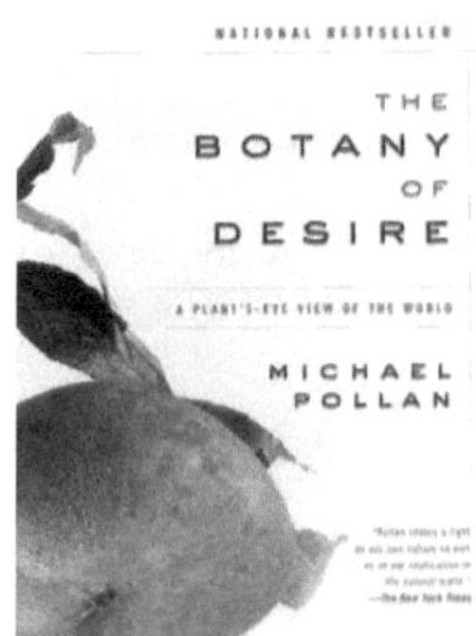

Blackstone carried apple seeds ("pips") with him & planted an orchard on Beacon Hill in Boston.

43). In **1623, William Blackstone**, an English clergyman, was credited with planting the first apple trees in Boston.

BLAXTON'S YELLOW SWEETING

Blaxton cultivated and named the first variety of American apples, the Yellow Sweeting.

44). Later, **in 1635,** he planted an apple orchard in Rhode Island, and he is thought by some to have introduced America's **first native apple** variety, **Blaxton's Yellow Sweeting.**

45). Another portion of the crop was cut and pressed into apple **juice,** which then fermented naturally into hard apple cider and was consumed year-round by the whole family.

46). Some of the hard apple cider could ferment further in air to produce apple cider vinegar and this was used as a natural medicine, as a condiment.

47). Apple Cider Vinegar was used for preserving liquid for fresh vegetables as well as for a condiment.

48). During the first half of the **nineteenth century,** John Chapman (aka **c**) became a folk hero by sharing apple seeds with frontier settlers and planting many of them himself from Pennsylvania, where he operated a nursery in the Susquehanna valley, all the way westward to Ohio and Indiana.

49). During the labor-intensive haying and harvesting season, American farmers in the eighteenth and **nineteenth centuries** would drink apple cider vinegar as a refreshing and energizing tonic. Often the vinegar was diluted with fruit juice known as "**switchels**".

SWITCHELS

Switchel is composed of ginger-water or haymaker's punch is a drink made of water mixed with vinegar, and/or seasoned with ginger. It is usually sweetened with molasses, though honey, sugar, brown sugar, or maple syrup are sometimes used instead.

50). Because of its usefulness and availability, apple cider and apple cider vinegar became a common **unit of exchange,** especially in rural areas where currency was relatively scarce.

51). It's no wonder therefore, that many farmers produced more apple cider and apple cider vinegar than they required, then used the extra **to pay for local services** such as those provided by doctors, teachers, and the clergy.

52). By 1817, the American Pomologist, William Coxe reported that **apple cider** in the mid-Atlantic states was selling for about **$5** per hogshead (63 gallons), **apple cider vinegar** was selling for $15 price.

AMERICAN POMOLOGIST, WILLIAM COXE & ACV

"William Coxe (1762-1831), a pomologist, was one of the foremost fruit growers in America who experimented with new varieties of fruits at his home in Burlington, New Jersey.

The study of **POMOLOGY** is the branch of botany that studies the **cultivation of fruit**.

NATURAL HAIR LOSS TREATMENT I

53). Apple cider vinegar (ACV) has long been used as a natural hair care product to promote healthy hair in both men and woman. Its **acidity** is close to that of natural hair, it's a good **conditioner** and **cleaning agent** and an effective **germ killer**

<u>Six Apple cider vinegar benefits for the hair:</u>

1.Vinegar hair rinse

2.Hair Herbal rinse

3.Essential oil vinegar hair rinse

4.Dandruff and itchy scalp relief

5.Natural hair loss treatment

6.Home Remedy for head Lice

54). <u>Hair Rinse</u>
Apple cider vinegar gets rid of residue build-up on hair, leaving it soft and shiny. Mix 1/2 cup apple cider vinegar with 1-quart water and use as a final rinse after shampooing.

55). <u>ACV Natural Hair Rinse –</u>
Hair is on the **mildly acidic** side of the pH scale and has an ideal pH of 4.5 to 5.5; an apple cider vinegar rinse has a pH of 2.9.Rinsing with apple cider vinegar will help **balance the pH** of your hair & remove the **buildup** from the use of styling products shampoos.

<u>**NATURAL HAIR LOSS TREATMENT II**</u>

56). <u>**Vinegar Hair Rinse: Natural Hair Care I**</u>

Rinsing will also close the numerous cuticle scales which cover and protect

The surface of each hair shaft. This imparts a smoother surface which

Reflects more light and as a result leaves your hair shinier,

Smoother and easier to manage.

<u>**NATURAL HAIR LOSS TREATMENT III**</u>

57). <u>Vinegar Hair Rinse: Natural Hair Care II</u>

Make your own healthy after-shampoo hair rinse by

Mixing 1/3 of a cup (75 ml) of ACV into

A quart (1 liter) of water.

You can then store this mixture in a plastic bottle

And keep it in the shower for ready use.

Apply the vinegar rinse after shampooing

And then rinse it all out,

Or for extra conditioning,

You can leave the rinse on your hair.

<u>**NATURAL HAIR LOSS TREATMENT III**</u>

58).<u>Hair Herbal Rinse – Natural Hair Care Product</u>

By infusing various **herbs** into the vinegar rinse, you can **enhance** different **hair colors** and **condition**

hair at the same time.

<u>Six herbs to use with ACV:</u>

1.For dark hair:.......Parsley, Rosemary, Sage
2.For light hair: .....Chamomile, Marigold
3.For red hair:.......Henna
4.For oily hair:...... Lavender, Thyme, Witch Hazel,
5.For dry hair:...... Marigold
6.For brittle hair...Horsetail

59). <u>Your own **herbal hair rinse** product</u>:
1. Place 2 tablespoons of the dried herb into a tea ball and put in a warmed tea pot.

2.Pour 1 pint (500 ml) of boiling water over the herbs and infuse for 2 hours.

3.Allow the liquid to cool then pour it into a quart (1 liter) jar & shake well.

4.Add 1 pint (500 ml) of apple cider vinegar, refrigerate and mix well.
To add extra **fragrance** to the herbal rinse, a few drops of lavender, lemon & rose.

60) <u>Essential oil vinegar hair rinse – Natural Hair</u>
A faster way to enhance the hair conditioning effect by making a batch, just add 5 drops of the

essential oil to 1 cup (250 ml) of apple cider vinegar. When you are ready to rinse your hair, take 1

tablespoon and 1 cup of warm water.

<u>(6) Essential Oils in a vinegar hair rinse:</u>
1.Lavender

2.Lemon

3.Rose

4.Rosemary

5.Sage

6.Lily of the Valley

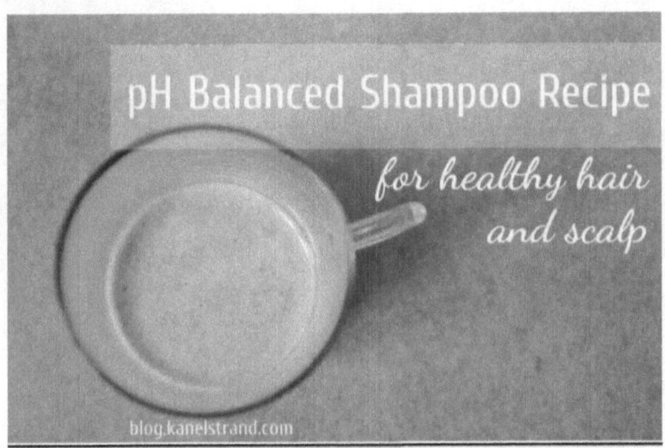

61). ACV KILLS BACTERIA

The acids and enzymes in ACV kill the **"bottle bacillus"**, a bacteria that is one of the causes for many scalp and hair conditions such as dandruff, itchy scalp, hair loss and often baldness. The bacteria clogs hair follicles allowing dry crusts to form that itch and flake. For a simple home treatment for dandruff and itchy scalp, apply full strength **ACV to the scalp**, rub in, and leave on for a half hour to an hour before washing your hair. For an **extra strength** natural hair care product, apple cider vinegar can be infused with herbs such as stinging nettle, southernwood, goose grass, plantain and burdock root all of which help prevent dandruff on their own.

ACV TO THE SCALP

This process is used to treat all scalp problems that include dry scalp, itchy scalp, dry itchy scalp, dry and dandruff, itchy and dandruff, scalp buildup, scalp psoriasis and flaky scalp

<u>**NATURAL HAIR LOSS TREATMENT IV**</u>

APPLE CIDER VINEGAR- MIRACLE HEALTH SYSTEM FOR NATURAL HAIR LOSS TREATMENT:

62). <u>Bald and thinning areas</u>
Apply to scalp an hour before shampooing- 2 Tbsp ACV mixed with a tiny pinch cayenne. powder.
Before bed, mix a royal jelly capsule with one tsp ACV, pat on bald areas

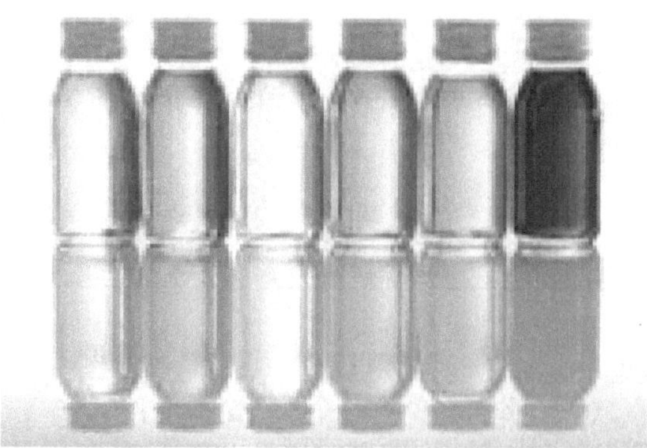

63). <u>Healthy Hair Rinse</u>

Given above and apply it full strength to the scalp. Rub it in and leave it on for a half hour to an hour
before washing your hair.

64). <u>Dandruff Treatment</u>

Simply pour a few Tbsp of vinegar on your hair, massage into your scalp, then rinse & wash hair.
Make your own vinegar mixture as per the mixture above.

65). <u>Improve hair quality</u>

Mix 1 cup of vinegar and warm water into a large glass and use to rinse your hair after you shampoo.
Vinegar adds highlights to brunette hair, restores the acid mantel & removes soap film and sebum oil.

66). <u>Clean Hairbrush</u>
Clean a hairbrush by soaking in a white distilled vinegar sore contagious and an intense itching.

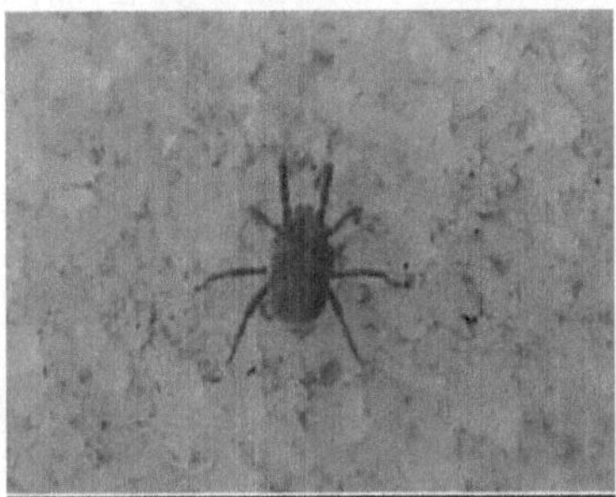

NATURAL HAIR TREATMENT LICE V

67. <u>Allergic reaction</u>
ACV acts as a toxin for the saliva in the mouth of lice.

68). <u>If you find that</u> **commercial** <u>lice</u> preparations are **too toxic** (many contain pesticides) for you or your child's skin, try the following herbal head louse treatment described in the Gale Encyclopedia of Alternative Medicine that uses all-natural hair care products: Carefully brush the child's head with a mixture of 3 parts olive oil and 1-part lavender essential oil.

1.First apply to a small area to test for allergic sensitivity or skin reaction.
2.The hair should be saturated with the olive oil mixture and a shower cap put on for 5 hours.
3.The olive oil clogs the breathing pores of lice and they can't hold their breath longer than 4 hours.

Follow this by an **apple cider vinegar rinse** to unglue the nits from the hair. Nits or lice eggs are small and can be pearly to grey in color. Then, using a fine-tooth comb, parents should comb the child's hair meticulously to remove the lice eggs from the hair shaft. And finally, wash the child's hair with a natural shampoo. Once completed, check the child's hair every other day for the next 10 days, and if needed repeat the treatment.

It is also helpful when children get lice, if you take warm vinegar and put it on the hair also take your nit comb and dip it in the vinegar. As you run it through the hair it helps remove the nits. It is supposed to be able to help break down the glue the nits use to stay attached to the hair.

VINEGAR OUTDOORS

Vinegar can be used in many wonderful ways outside your home. Vinegar is a great alternative to toxic chemicals for controlling weeds, pests, and disease in your yard. For example, vinegar (particularly apple cider vinegar) is a key ingredient in organic herbicides and fertilizers. This article includes various hints on how you can use vinegar with outdoors activities and maintenance projects.

THE GARDEN IS WHERE VINEGAR CAN DO WONDERS.

69). Camping Equipment
When you are camping, you need to do more than one thing. Vinegar should be on that list.

70). Camping/Hiking
Add several drops of vinegar to a canteen or insulated container of water.

71). Clean Cement Pond
Cure a cement pond before adding fish & plants by adding 1 gallon of vinegar to 200 gallons of water.

72). Catch Moths
To catch moths, use a mixture of 2 parts vinegar & 1-part molasses. Place mixture & hang on a tree.

73)   Clean outdoor pump
When cleaning outdoor fountain, soak the pump in distilled vinegar to remove any mineral deposits.

74).   Cleaning plastic
Plastic tarps or outdoor equipment coverings can be made antistatic by cleaning them with a solution of 1 tablespoon vinegar to 1-gallon water. This may also reduce the amount of dust.

75). Cleaning canvas
To clean canvas tents or other canvas materials, dip a bristle scrub brush in warm water, spray on the cleaner, and brush. If your tent develops mildew, clean by wiping them with vinegar & dry in the sun.

76). Clean your car
Use it full-strength to polish car chrome with a cloth and see it shine! Use it on your car's windshield.

77). Polish car chrome
Apply vinegar full strength to the chrome with cloth

78). Keep car windows frost free
When you must leave your car outside overnight in the winter, mix 3 parts vinegar to 1-part water and coat the windows with this solution; This will keep windshields ice and frost-free.

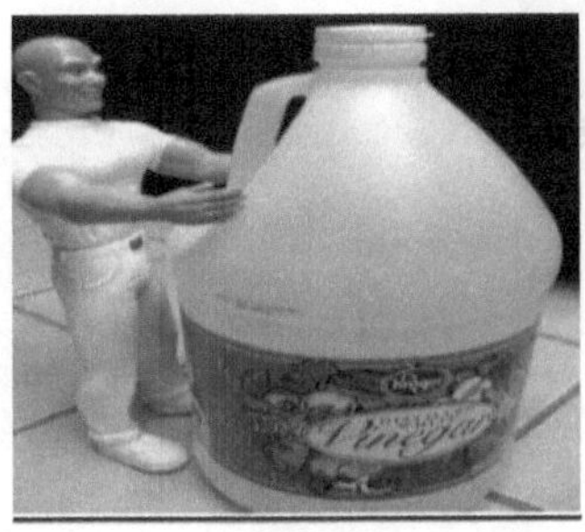

FOR EVERYDAY HOUSEHOLD USES I

HOUSEHOLD CLEANING I

79). Septic Tanks
If you have a septic tank, use vinegar instead of harsh chemicals to clean the toilet bowl. Let it set overnight if you can; it will help keep germs down.

80). Clean a toilet bowl
Pour in one cup of White Vinegar, let it stand for 5 minutes, and flush.

81). Reduce mineral deposits in pipes
Use a spray bottle or mister filled with a solution of 50/50 Heinz Vinegar & water around door jambs, window sills and water pipes.

82). Clean rust from tools and bolts
Soak the rusted tool or bolt in undiluted vinegar overnight

83). Loosen a rusted screw or a rusted lock
Simply pour some vinegar on or into the area and leave for a short while

84). Clean plastic
Plastic can be cleaned and made anti-static by wiping down with a solution of 1 tablespoon of distilled vinegar to 1 gallon of water. This will cut down on the plastics' tendency to attract dust

85). <u>Replenish your carpets</u>
Use diluted 1:1 in water to take pet odors out of carpets. Find the spot and saturate it with about 1 1/2 times the original volume. Let set for a while then blot up. Repeat if necessary, for large spots.

86). <u>Remove carpet stains</u>
A mixture of one teaspoon of liquid detergent and 1 teaspoon of distilled vinegar in a pint of lukewarm water will remove non-oily stains from carpets. Rinse with a towel moistened with clean water and blot dry. Repeat this until the stain is gone.

87). <u>Freshen up the washing machine</u>
Clean the hoses and unclog soap scum. Once a month pour one cup of vinegar into the washing machine and run the machine through a normal cycle, without clothes

88). <u>Blankets</u>: When washing cotton or washable wool blankets, add 2 cups of vinegar to the last rinse cycle. This will help remove the soap and make blankets soft and fluffy.

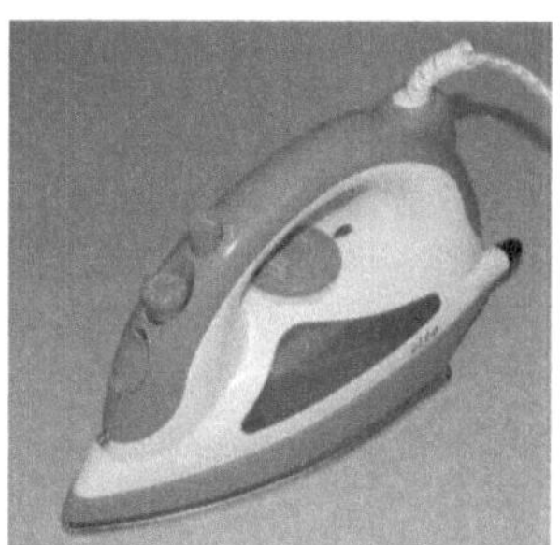

89). <u>**Unclog a steam iron**</u>
Unclog a steam iron by pouring equal amounts of vinegar and water into the iron's water chamber. Turn to steam and leave the iron on for 5 minutes in an upright position. Any loose particles should come out.

90).   Clean a scorched iron
Clean a scorched iron plate by heating equal parts of vinegar and salt in a small pan. Then rub the solution on the cooled iron surface to remove burned stains

91).   Remove Scorch Marks on Clothes
Rub lightly with Heinz White Vinegar, then wipe.

92).   Remove stains from chinaware
Mixture of salt and vinegar will clean coffee and tea stains from chinaware

93). Clean china and glassware
Clean china and fine glassware by adding a cup of vinegar to a sink of warm water. Gently dip the glass/china in the solution and let dry.

94). Clean Can Opener
Clean the wheel of a can opener using white distilled vinegar and an old toothbrush.

95). Prevent soapy film on glassware
Place a cup of White Vinegar on the bottom rack of your dishwasher, run for five minutes, then run though the full cycle.

96). Shine brass
Brass, copper and pewter will shine if cleaned with the following mixture. Dissolve 1 teaspoon of salt in 1 cup of distilled vinegar.

97). Shine Copper
On heavily tarnished copper or copper-alloy to be cleaned up, use a paste made of salt and vinegar.

98). Clean your piano keys –
Clean piano keys with a solution of equal parts vinegar and water. Dip a soft cloth into the solution and ring out as much as possible. Wipe each key gently, drying with a soft cloth as you go.

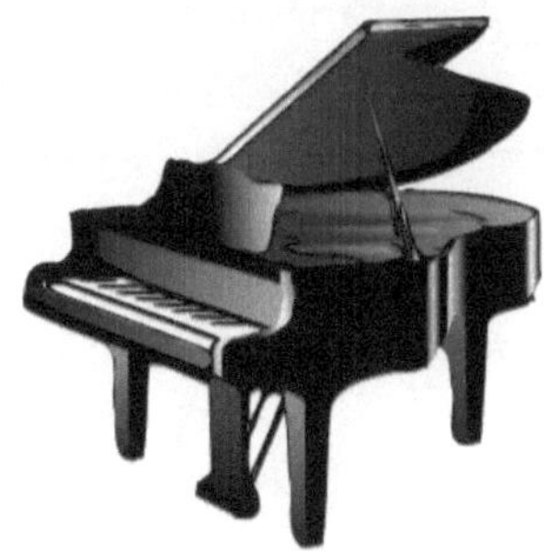

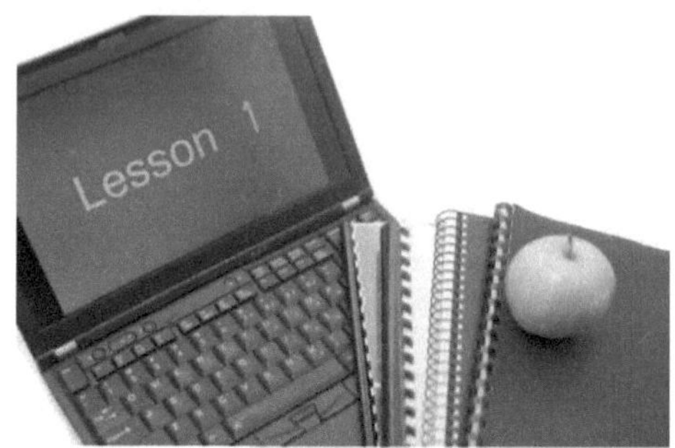

99).   Clean Your Computer

Vinegar has several elements which make it a good cleanser. It has a well-known ability to disinfect. You can clean your computer by mixing 50/50, water & vinegar in a bucket.

100).   Clean Your Printer

Add equal parts vinegar and water. Turn off all the components and mix equal parts of vinegar and water in a bucket. Wet a cloth in the solution and ring it out. Make sure that the cloth is not dripping wet, as you do not want water to fall into the interior of your keyboard or computer.

101).   Clean Your Fax Machine

Wipe all the surfaces of your electronics and get them shining clean. Use cotton swabs around small or tough to reach areas, for example, in between the keys of the keyboard

102).   Clean your scissors –

Instead of washing your scissors with water, which will likely just rust the fastener, wipe them clean with a cloth dipped in full strength vinegar then dry them off with a clean, dry cloth.

103).   Clean stainless steel

Clean stainless steel by wiping with a vinegar dampened cloth
1
04).   Clean Exhaust Fans

Wipe grease off exhaust fan grids, the inside of your oven, or anywhere grease gathers with a sponge soaked in white vinegar.

105).   Cleaning Grills

To make cleaning the grill easier, spray a solution of half water and half white vinegar on the cooking surface.

106).Peeling off cement floors
First paint the floor with white vinegar. Once it is dry, apply the paint.

107).Peeling off galvanized metal
First paint the metal with white vinegar. Once it is dry, apply the paint

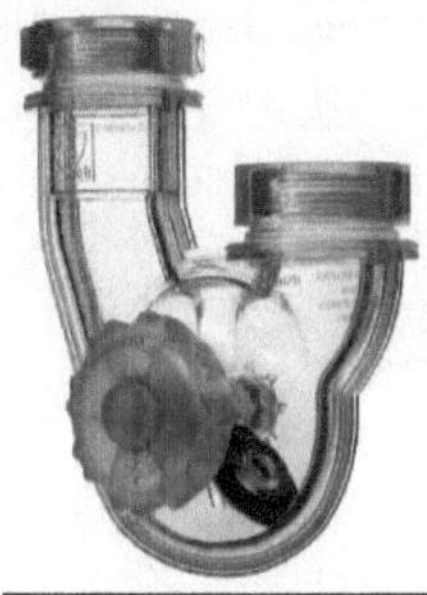

108). Unclog a Drain
Pour a handful of baking soda down the drain and add 1/2 cup of vinegar. Rinse with hot water

109). Keep fruit flies away from a jar
Pour 1/2 inch of cider vinegar in the bottom of a small jar and punch a dozen or so holes in the lid (using an ice pick). The vinegar attracts the flies through the holes, and they can't get out.

110). Keep flies away from a bowl
Or just set out a dish with the vinegar plus a few drops of dish detergent. It attracts & drowns them

111). Flies around the pool
Pour vinegar around the sides of your pool; it helps keeps flies away.

112). Shine your linoleum
No-wax linoleum will shine better if wiped with 1/2 cup of white vinegar in 1/2 gallon of water

113). Vinyl Floors
Add 1/2 cup vinegar to a gal. of water to keep your vinyl no wax floors clean and shining.

114).Better steam cleaning
Use vinegar in the steam cleaner to reduce bubbles

115). Clean wood better
Mix vinegar with linseed oil and use it to clean wood

116). Clean eye glasses
Clean your eye glasses by wiping each lens with a drop of vinegar

EVERYDAY OUTSIDE USES I (

117). <u>Prolong the life of lantern wicks</u>
Soak new propane lantern wicks in vinegar for 3 hours. Let dry before using. Will burn brighter.

118). <u>Deter ants</u> around windows
Spray vinegar around door and window frames, under appliances, and along other known ant trails.

119). <u>Deter ants around points of entry</u>
You may be able to stop a troop of ants from marching into your house if you can identify their points of entry and wipe areas with undiluted vinegar, near sinks.

120). <u>Anthills</u>
Eliminate anthills by pouring in white vinegar.

121). <u>Natural air deodorizer</u>

Air freshener, used with baking soda - use 1 teaspoon baking soda, 1 tablespoon vinegar and 2 cups of water. After it stops foaming, mix well & use in a (recycled) spray bottle into the air.

122). <u>Remove cigarette smells</u>
Deodorize a room filled with cigarette smoke or paint fumes. Place a small bowl White Vinegar.

123). <u>Fix sagging cane chairs</u>
To improve the seats of sagging cane chairs, sponge them with a hot solution of half vinegar and half water. Place the chairs out in the hot sun to dry

124). <u>Remove bumper stickers</u>
Vinegar mixed with salt. It cleans copper, bronze, brass, dishes, pots, pans, skillets, glasses and windows, Remove decals/bumper stickers by soaking a cloth in Vinegar several minutes .

125). <u>Cleaner windows</u>
Mix vinegar with water or simply spray full-strength on glass and mirrors or wipe windows dry with crumpled-up newspapers.

126). <u>Eliminate mildew and dust</u>
Eliminate mildew, wipe walls with ACV.

127). <u>Cleaning coolers</u>
Picnic jugs & coolers have musty smells. Rinse with undiluted vinegar, wash with soap and water.

128). <u>Remove fizzy drink stains</u>
Spots caused by cola-based soft drinks can be removed by sponging vinegar directly onto the stain .

129). <u>Eliminate dust from Air conditioner blades</u>
Sponging away grease and dirt with a sponge dipped in distilled vinegar will keep exhaust fans.

130). Clean fireplace bricks
Clean fireplace bricks with vinegar to remove soot.

131). Remove price tags or stickers
Paint them with several coats of vinegar and let it soak in, they'll either slide off easily or require a little heavier rubbing

132). Remove old chewing gum
Remove chewing gum from carpets by applying hot vinegar to the gum. The gum should dissolve. You can saturate the area with vinegar or heat, it will work faster.

134). Remove old glue
To loosen old glue around rungs and joints of tables and chairs under repair, apply distilled vinegar with a small oil can or spray bottle.

135). You can use vinegar to remove wall paper.
First remove top layer of wallpaper. Then spray vinegar on and let set for a minute or two. Then pull backing away. Scrape excess glue off wall. Wipe remaining glue off with vinegar, rinse with water.

136). Shine leather
Give patent leather shoes and bags a better shine by wiping them down with white distilled vinegar.

137). Clean leather
Clean leather with a mixture of 1 cup boiled linseed oil and 1 cup vinegar. Carefully apply, . Let dry.

138). Clean Pain brushes
Boil the paint brush in vinegar, or soak it in very hot vinegar, then wash in soapy water

139). Room freshener
To add a pleasant scent to a room while at the same time removing an unpleasant smell, add cardamom or other fragrant spice to a bowl of ACV.

140). Furniture Polish
You can make furniture polish with 1-part vinegar & 3 parts lemon oil.

141). Replenish dull wood
Varnished wood often takes on a cloudy appearance. it can be removed by rubbing the wood with a cloth from a solution of 1 tbsp. of vinegar.

142).Clean dirty wood
Dirt and grime can be easily removed with a solution of 1 cup of ammonia, 1/2 cup of distilled vinegar & 1/4 cup of baking soda.

143. Remove stubborn glass rings
Stubborn rings may be removed by rubbing with a mixture of equal parts of distilled vinegar and olive oil. Rub with the grain and polish.

144). Calcium deposit build-up
Vinegar is great for removing calcium deposit build up. Use full strength and allow to saturate. Time depends on condition.

145). Clean drinking glasses
Soaking cloudy drinking glasses in warmed white vinegar for a few hours to remove the film, simply wipe clean, rinse, and dry.

146). Replenish wood paneling
Wood paneling may be cleaned with a mixture of 1 ounce of olive oil and 2 ounces of distilled vinegar in 1 quart of warm water.

147). Retard Patching Plaster
Add one tablespoon white vinegar to the water when mixing plaster to slow the drying time.

148). Removes smoke stains from walls
To remove nicotine from walls before painting, always use vinegar in hot water. Will remove stains and will not bleed through the paint.

149). Wallpaper remover
Mix equal parts Vinegar and hot water, Use a paint roller to wet the paper mixture. Repeat necessary.

150). Remove paint from glass
Soften hardened paint on glass by rubbing with undiluted vinegar.

151). Replenish sponges
To replenish a slimy sponge, soak the sponge in vinegar & water.

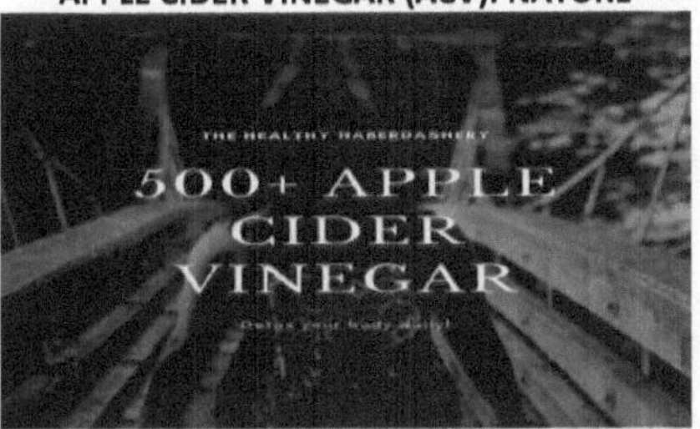

WORLD'S FIRST NATURAL CURE I

152). <u>Memory Improvement</u>
Drinking my Arthritis Cocktail will clear brain fog.

153). <u>Soothe a bee, mosquito or jellyfish sting</u>
Use a cotton ball to dab the irritated area with Vinegar straight from the bottle to relieve itching

154. <u>Respiratory problems</u>
To clear up respiratory congestion, inhale a vapor mist containing water and spoonsful of vinegar

155. <u>Reduce Anxiety Attacks</u>
Mix 570ml of cider vinegar with a bunch of picked lavender. Leave the mixture in an open bowl.

156. <u>Eliminate hiccups</u>
You take 1 tablespoon full and swallow when you have the hiccups. It stops them instantly! Cure the hiccups. Mix one teaspoon Apple Cider Vinegar in one cup of warm water, and drink.

157. <u>Acid indigestion</u>
Mix a solution of vinegar and honey in equal measures. Take 1 teaspoon of the mixture before drinking a cup of hot water. Repeat daily.

158. <u>Relief from asthma</u>
Add a tablespoon of cider vinegar to a glass of water and take regular sips from the glass to help reduce the wheezing. Repeat as needed.

159. <u>Relieve dizziness</u>
Mix two teaspoons of cider vinegar and two teaspoons of honey into a glass of water and drink a glass (3X) three times a day to relieve dizziness; My Apple Cider Vinegar Cocktail!

160. <u>Relieve sunburn</u>
Soak a washcloth in vinegar and gently apply it to sunburned skin for cool relief. Reapply to evaporates and re-hydrate sunburned skin.

161).Make a good liniment
To make a good liniment, beat 1 whole egg, add 1 cup of vinegar, 1 cup of turpentine and blend the mixture. Apply with a sponge.

162). Reduce Nausea
To reduce the general feeling of sickness, take a teaspoon of clove vinegar in addition to: My Apple Cider Vinegar Cocktail!

163). Soothe an upset stomach
Cure an upset stomach by drinking two teaspoons of Apple Cider Vinegar in one cup of water: My Apple Cider Vinegar Cocktail!

164).Treat ringworm
Apply undiluted cider vinegar directly to the affected skin areas several times during the day

165). Relieve dry and itchy skin
Add 2 tablespoons to bath water up to 1 cup, add just before bathing.

166). Eliminate constipation
A regular intake of cider vinegar will promote regular bowel movements & constipation: My Apple Cider Vinegar Cocktail!

167). Treat colitis
Mix two teaspoons of cider vinegar and two teaspoons of honey into a glass of water and drink a glass three times a day to treat colitis

168). Relief from shingles
To relieve the pain and itching associated with shingles, dab undiluted vinegar onto the affected area.

169). Fight dandruff
Rinse hair with vinegar and 2 cups of warm water after shampooing

170). Weight loss
Vinegar naturally helps to remove fat from the body - apple cider vinegar is especially good for this. Drink some in a glass of water a few times a day & add a little honey to reduce your appetite: Try My Apple Cider Vinegar Cocktail!

171). Soothe a sore throat
Put a teaspoon of vinegar in a glass of water. Gargle and then swallow or use for vinegar is to use 1 tablespoon vinegar to an 8-ounce glass of warm water for a sore throat. Gargle with 2 mouthfuls.

172). Cure for colds
Mix one-quarter cup Apple Cider Vinegar with one-quarter cup honey. Take one tbsp. 6 to 8 times daily; My Apple Cider Vinegar Cocktail!

173).   Remove cold sores quicker
To help dry and out the cold sore, dab the affected area with gauze soaked in diluted white vinegar.
Sorry,   but it will probably sting a little

174). Promote blood clotting
Add two tablespoons of cider vinegar to a glass of water and drink a glass several times a day to
promote the thickening of blood

175).Aids diarrhea
Add a teaspoon of cider vinegar to a glass of water and drink before meals. You can also supplement
with another glass between meals,

176). Quench your thirst
Drink unfiltered apple cider vinegar mixed with cold water and sweeten to your taste. (honey or stevia
(diabetes: My Apple Cider Vinegar Cocktail! (Quick recipe)

177). Treat chest colds
Add 1/4 cup or more vinegar to the vaporizer, cover head with a towel & breathe. Also try: My Apple
Cider Vinegar Cocktail!

178). Fast relief for skin burns
For fast skin burn relief, apply ice cold vinegar cubes right away. This should prevent burn blisters and
relieve the stinging.

179). Faster Relief for Skin burns
Soak a piece of clean cloth in chilled vinegar and apply it to the burn. Repeat the process every 15
minutes until pain subsides.

180). **<u>PROMOTE BURN HEALING I</u>**

Apply un-pasteurized apple cider vinegar with the

aid of a soft cotton ball, directly to **burns** or **skin**

Great for clearing up of acne

Will provide soothing to your face

and massage into the rest of

the torso of the body

to promote rapid healing

without scarring.

181). <u>Instant Relief for burns</u>.
Stove and oil burns are instantly relieved and used as an antiseptic.

182). <u>Soften gallstones</u>
A regular intake of cider vinegar is beneficial to the breaking up gallstones and kidney stones.

183).<u>Relieve hay fever</u>
Mix two teaspoons of cider vinegar and two teaspoons of honey into a glass of water and drink a glass three times a day during the hay fever season for relief from this annoying problem.

184).<u>Prevent ulcers</u>
A regular intake of cider vinegar will help to prevent ulcers: My Apple Cider Vinegar Cocktail!

185). <u>Beat insomnia</u>
Beat insomnia the natural way by taking a mixture of two teaspoons of cider vinegar and two teaspoons of honey in water before bed.

186). <u>Clean dentures</u>
Clean dentures Soak dentures overnight in White Vinegar, then brush away tartars, then smile.

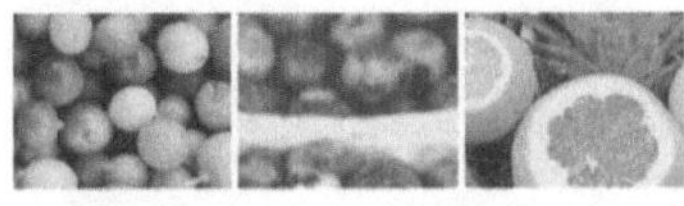

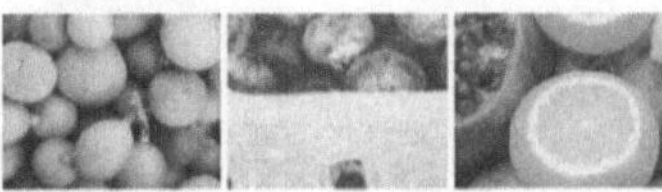

PROMOTE HEALING I

187). <u>Cough relief</u>
Relieve a cough by mixing one-half cup Apple Cider Vinegar, one-half cup water, one teaspoon cayenne pepper and four teaspoons honey.

188). <u>Relieve Chronic Fatigue</u>
Mix three teaspoons of cider vinegar with one cup of honey and take at night before going to bed to overcome tiredness during the day. Especially effective: My Apple Cider Vinegar Cocktail!

189). <u>Refreshing Bath</u>
Add lavender vinegar to your bath water for the perfect tonic.

190). <u>Eliminate cramps</u>
Mix a teaspoon of honey, a teaspoon of cider vinegar and a tablespoon of calcium lactate together; take a teaspoon once a day, i.e.: My Apple Cider Vinegar Cocktail!

191). <u>Relieve aching feet</u>
For the perfect foot bath, mix 1/2 cup of cider vinegar with 2 quarts water while sipping: My Apple Cider Vinegar Cocktail!

192).<u>Relieve stiff muscles</u>
A regular intake of cider vinegar will help to break down the lactic acid that can make muscles painful. Try, My Apple Cider Vinegar Cocktail!

193). <u>Reduce high blood pressure</u>
Take a daily mixture of two teaspoons of cider vinegar and two teaspoons of honey in a glass of water to help reduce blood pressure. Try, My Apple Cider Vinegar Cocktail!

194). <u>Alleviate headaches</u>
Soak a handkerchief in white vinegar hold against the nostrils for a few minutes, taking deep breaths to inhale the aroma of the vinegar

195). <u>Relieve toothache</u>

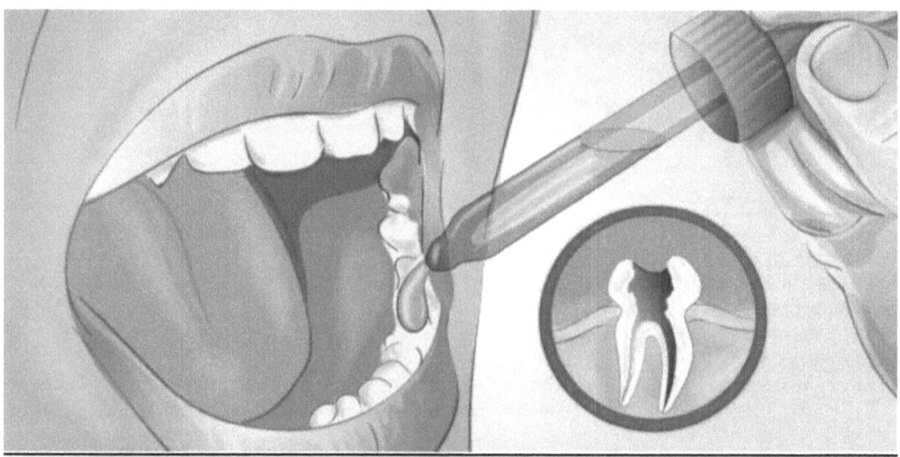

In times of desperation, try a hot mouth wash with a teaspoon of white vinegar added to the water, holding in mouth will deaden pain.

196. <u>Diffusing Calcium Build-up</u>

When taking calcium-magnesium tablets/or powder, wash it down with something acidic (like vinegar diluted in water), so that it will dissolve the cal-magnesium, then your body can assimilate it.

197). <u>Poison Ivy</u>

Our grandmother's swore by vinegar as an antiseptic from abrasions to reduce itch, poison ivy, and mosquito bites.

198). Cat Allergies
Apple cider vinegar will take certain allergies away. You can now have an indoor cat without worrying about allergies.

199). Lessens Stunted Growth
Paul C. Bragg made over 10 scientific health expeditions, studying the growth of various races of people. He found areas where the topsoil was deficient in Potassium, people were prone to be stunted.

200). Spastic Colon
Drinking My Arthritis Apple Cider Vinegar can improve a Spastic Colon as it will melt the acid crystals that cause the painful colons.

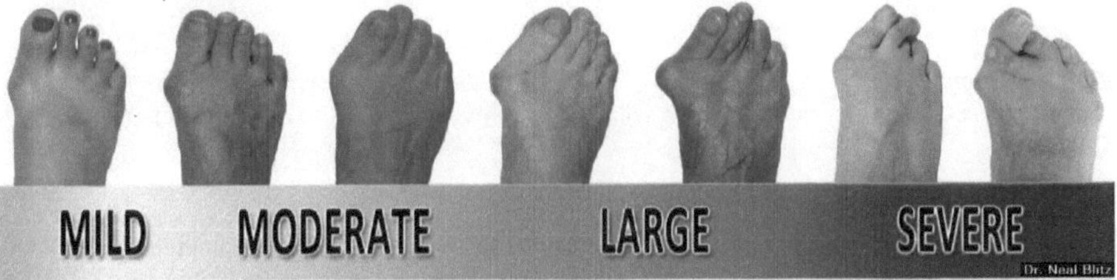

201). Overall
My Arthritis Apple cider vinegar can be consumed at least 3x day. It can be applied as an apple cider Vinegar compress 1) Place a Thin ACV soaked cloth over the throat 2) cover with Saran Wrap 3) Use hot water bag.

202).Lung Congestion
Use Same compress listed above and gargle with Apple Cider Vinegar and water in a glass 3X day to remove any body toxins being eliminated through the throat tissues.

203). Heart Strengthening
Apple Cider Vinegar contains a natural chemical that combines with the heart fuel to make the heart muscle stronger and normalizing blood pressure. **Drink: My Apple Cider Vinegar Cocktail!**

204). Gallbladder Flush
For 2 days no food is to be eaten, only liquids. Combine in a glass: 1/3 Bragg's Olive Oil, 2/3 apple Juice & 1 tsp Bragg's Organic Apple Cider Vinegar. Drink 3X day and sleep on the right side pulling right knee up to chest to open pathway. **Drink: My Apple Cider Vinegar Cocktail!**

205).**ARTHRITIS COCKTAIL SHORTCUT** ;
Start with ½ gallon of Raw Apple Cider Juice, add ½ cup Apple Cider Vinegar. Shake in a jug, continue to add 1 tsp. of ACV.

206). Stiff Neck
For a stiff neck, take a half cup of vinegar in a warm water solution and soak a cloth in it, wrap it around your neck. Put a layer of plastic wrap (to keep your sheets dry).

207). Homemade Facial
Mix a "toner" using ½   water, 1/2 vinegar and a few aspirins. The acids in the vinegar force your old skin cells to flake off, like "alpha hydroxyl" products.

208). Perfume Odor
To remove the odor of a perfume you don't like. Just apply vinegar sprayed to get rid of perfume.

209). Belly Piercing Woes
To cure an infected belly button, warm some vinegar and dab it on the belly button until the infection clears!

210). Nose Piercing Woes
Nose piercing using vinegar can be used it for daily cleaning. Using vinegar in a pinch for daily cleaning, or spot infections could help.

211). Hangovers
A grandmother from Scotland used vinegar extensively on a cloth placed on her forehead to stop hangover headaches!

212). Smoke Detectors
Vinegar in a towel, twirled about the head will quickly stop the smoke detectors from screaming. It also freshens the air and captures the smoke smell before the whole house is caught on fire.

<u>FOOLPROOF WALL CLEARNER</u>

213). <u>Sure Fire Wall Cleaner</u>

This from a column in a newspaper... :

1 GALLON OF WATER

1 CUP BOTTLED AMMONIA

1/2 CUP BOTTLED VINEGAR

1/4 CUP BAKING SODA

Put the ammonia, vinegar and baking soda

Into the bucket of water.

STIR TO MIX THOROUGHLY.

Wash the walls from the bottom up for if or

Leaves marks that are very difficult

If not impossible to remove.

(This caution was printed in the paper along with the solution recipe).

214).   Super infected Athletes Foot Problem

Before bedtime soak the infected foot in apple cider vinegar. It will smell for a few seconds while disinfecting. Then, moisten gauze with apple cider vinegar and put it on the infection, binding it in place with an Ace bandage and covering it with a sock (rinsed in vinegar). Keep it on overnight & repeat until infection clears up.

215).   Headache Headband

Soak a while handkerchief in vinegar, wring it out, roll it up and tie it around the forehead.

216).   Ringworm with Pennies

Put a copper penny in vinegar and keep it there until it turns green.   Then take the wet penny & rub it on the ringworm. Repeat 3X a day.

217).   Super Wart Remover

Dab apple cider vinegar on the wart before it dries, then put baking soda on. Dust off the soda after 15 min., 6 times a day until gone.

218).   Yellow Jacket Repellent

When picnicking you can pour apple cider vinegar in saucers, place them around the area to ward off any unwelcome flying guests.

219).   Facial Neuralgia

Drinking My Arthritis Cocktail, ½ glass in 7 doses a day will help alleviate this problem over time and cleanse the overall system.

220).   Fevers

Enhance the properties of chicken soup by adding 1 tbsp vinegar, 1 crushed clove & a few drops of hot pepper sauce to the broth.

221).   Relieve Congestion

Try my Arthritis Cocktail and you'll be amazed at your calm stomach.

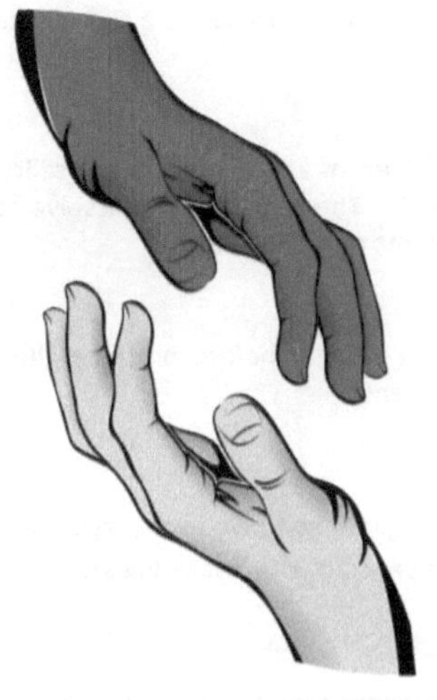

222). <u>Increases Blood Circulation</u>
Science tells us that ACV promotes blood circulation in the small blood capillaries that irrigate the skin. It is also antiseptic, combating yeasts, viruses, and bacteria that can cause infection.

223). <u>Maintains pH Balance</u>
Apple cider vinegar is rich in alpha-hydroxyl acids, helping to dissolve fatty deposits on the skin's surface and reducing scaly conditions, promoting a softer, smoother appearance; regulates skin's ph.

MAINTAINING PH BALANCE

Many doctors stress the importance of reducing acidity and increasing alkalinity with an alkaline diet because a balanced pH helps protect us from the inside out. Disease and disorder, they say, cannot take root in a body whose pH is in balance

224). <u>Facial spritzer</u>
Mix 1/2 apple cider vinegar and 1/2 water into a spray bottle. Very refreshing when sprayed on the face to relieve tiredness.

225). Overall Skin Cleanser
You can dilute 50/50, vinegar and pure water to use as a skin cleanser as most soaps are too alkaline to balance the Skin ph.

226). Super Anti-Acne Solution
Use ACV as an anti-acne solution. A lot of acne products use salicylic acid, which is basically aspirin with a few small chemical differences. The aspirin won't dissolve completely, but it works especially well against those big, deep acne spots older people get.

227). Disinfecting Toothbrush after onions
Dipping a wet toothbrush in white vinegar before brushing the teeth will help any bad breath, especially after eating onions & whitens.

228). For Softer .body
In your bathwater, add ½ cup of vinegar or so to warm the bath water when bathing and get double benefits – softer skin and a cleaner bathtub with less wring around the bath tub!

229). For softer hands
Spray your hands with a mist of vinegar or dip them in vinegar after washing dishes or soaping them in water to keep your hands soft.

230).   Treat liver spots
Mix a solution of one-part onion juice to two parts vinegar and run onto the affected area several times a day. It could take several weeks before any results are to be seen

231)   Lightening age Spots
Lightening age spots: Dab areas with straight apple cider vinegar overnight, sleep with gloves on for hands.

232). Fading Age Spots
Mix equal parts of onion juice & vinegar, use it daily on age spots. It works just like its expensive counterpart.

233). Eliminate hair loss
Add a teaspoon of cider vinegar to a glass of water, drink before each meal with another glass between meals to maintain hair growth

234). <u>Toenail Fungus Treatment</u>
Soak your feet in a strong solution of vinegar and water at least daily to get rid of toenail fungus.

235). <u>Relieve Athlete's Foot</u>
Rinse feet with apple cider vinegar several times a day. In addition to this, soak clean socks in a mixture of 1-part vinegar to 5 parts water.

236). <u>Foot Odor</u>
Get rid of foot odor by washing feet well with antiseptic soap daily, then soaking them in undiluted cider vinegar for 10 minutes or so.

237). <u>Underarm Odor</u>
To prolong the effects of deodorant, apply apple vinegar to the armpits after showing & also after you apply your deodorant.

238). <u>Remove calluses</u>
Try soaking your feet in a combination of white vinegar and warm water nightly and watch your feet soften.

239). <u>Eliminate corns</u>
Remove corns by making a poultice of one crumbled piece of bread soaked in one-quarter cup Vinegar. Let poultice sit for half an hour, then apply to the corn and tape in place overnight.

240). <u>Another Corn remover</u>
Soak a piece of stale bread (a cloth would do as well) in vinegar, and tape it over the callus overnight.

241). <u>Callus Remover</u>: Apply vinegar with cotton ball on corns.

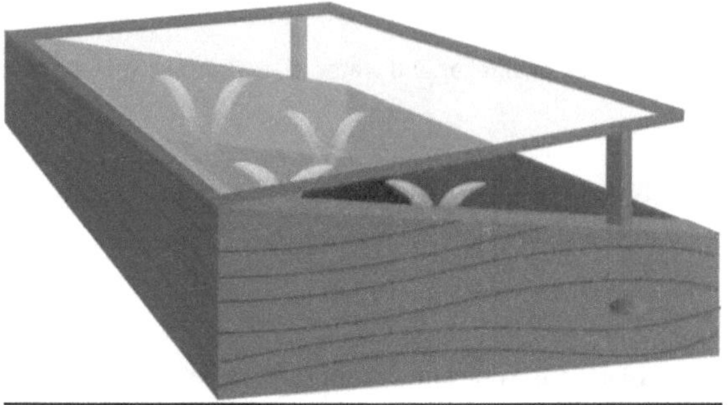

242). <u>Germination</u> of okra and asparagus seed by rubbing seeds between two pieces of sandpaper, then soak seeds overnight in a pint of warm water with ½ cup vinegar and a squirt of liquid disk soap

243). <u>Seeds</u>: Use without the sandpaper rub for seeds like nasturtium, parsley, beets, parsnips.

244). <u>Beans De-Gasser</u>

De-gas beans by adding Apple Cider Vinegar (1/8-1/4 c) to soaking water. Soak overnight, then rinse thoroughly. Add a little to the water when you cook them also. Works for split peas and garbanzos also.

BEANS DE-GASSER + HEALTH + APPLE CIDER VINEGAR

**Beans, though super nutritious, have a high concentration of
indigestible sugars and phytic acid that can wreak havoc on the digestive system.
ACV helps break down these stubborn starches.**

245). <u>Clean vegetables</u> by soaking them in a solution of vinegar and water (2 tablespoons to a gallon of water) to help remove chemical residues, pesticides and insects.

246). <u>Wilted vegetables</u>, add them to a pan of cold water to which 1 tablespoon of apple cider vinegar has been added. This will also help to destroy any undesirable microorganisms.

247).   <u>Steaming vegetables</u>, add 1 tablespoon of vinegar to the water used for steaming instead of table salt. The veggies will retain their bright colors and will not taste bland.

248.   <u>Dried beans are less gas producing</u> when eaten, add vinegar to the soaking water and then try cooking with vinegar. Vinegar helps to break down cellulose in any fibrous or stringy vegetables.

249).   <u>Preserve left over ginger root</u> in vinegar. First peel and slice or grate the ginger then place it in a glass jar, cover it with apple cider or balsamic vinegar and store in the refrigerator.

250).   <u>Clean cauliflower</u> by adding a spoonful of vinegar to water to make cauliflower white and clean.

FRUITS

251). <u>Clean fruits</u> by soaking them in a solution of vinegar and water (2 tablespoons to a gallon of water) to help remove chemical residues and insects.

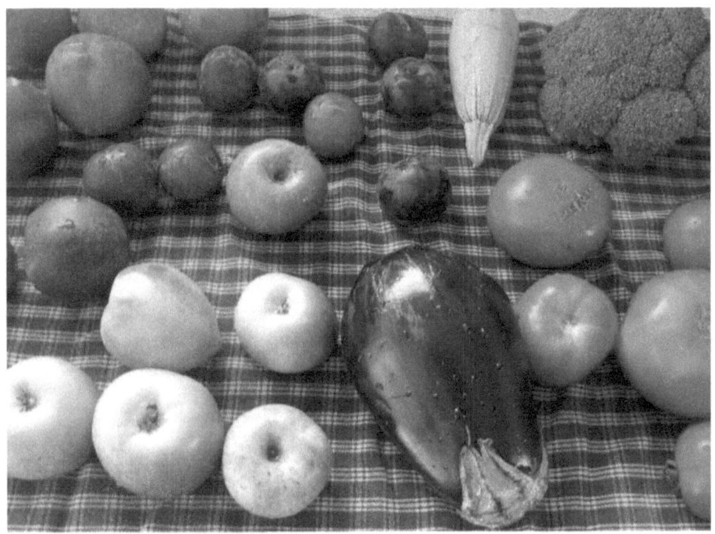

252).<u>Prevent cut and peeled fruits,</u> such as apples, from browning by placing the cut-up pieces into an apple cider vinegar solution (1 tablespoon ACV in the holding water) until they are ready to be used.

253).Adding 1 tablespoon of vinegar for every 2 1/2 cups of flour will help bread to rise. Reduce the

amount of water added by the same amount of vinegar added.

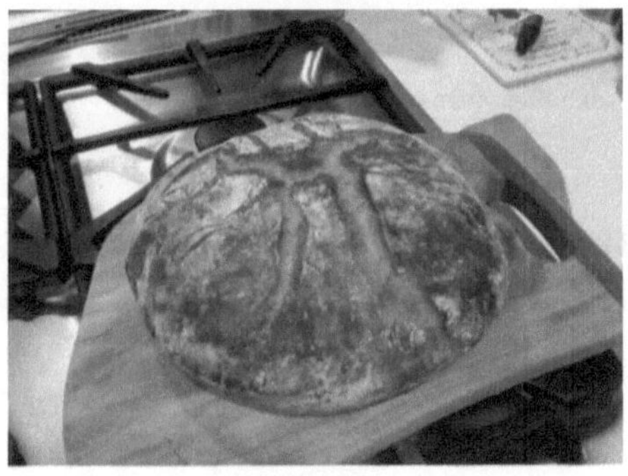

254).   To add luster to the crust of homemade bread, brush the top of the bread with vinegar two

minutes before it is done, then finish baking it in the oven.

255). Keep cheese from molding

Cheese can be kept soft and mold-free by wrapping it in a cloth saturated with vinegar and then keeping it in the refrigerator in an airtight container.

256). Boil better eggs

Boil better eggs by adding 2 tablespoons of vinegar to the water before boiling. This keeps them from cracking. When boiling eggs, add vinegar to the water to prevent white from leaking out of a cracked egg.

257) Hard boiled eggs add 1 or 2 tablespoons of vinegar to the cooking water to prevent leaking out.

258). Poached eggs,

Put vinegar in the poaching water will help the eggs keep their shape.

259). Potato Salad,
Stop yellowing after cutting potatoes, put in water & add a little vinegar.

260).   Egg substitute:

Put 1 tbsp of apple cider vinegar for each egg.

261).   Poach better eggs

When poaching eggs, add a teaspoon of vinegar to the water to prevent separation

262). Tenderize Meats
Tenderize meats by marinating them in a wine vinegar mixed with herbs. This will also enhance the meat flavor. Refrigerate to Marinate meat overnight.

263). Lessen Gamey flavor
To lessen the gamey flavor of wild meat, soak the meat in a vinegar-water solution prior to cooking.

264). Improve the Flavor
Improve the flavor and texture of boiled meat by cooking with vinegar by adding a tablespoon.

265). Meat Enhancer
Sage Vinegar adds flavoring to tenderize meats.

266). Marinate meat
On a different note, most meat marinades with vinegar can't hurt.

267. Improve the flavor of ham
Adding a little vinegar to your basting would give extra flavor and tenderness to a ham.

268). Cook better roasts
Marinating meat in vinegar kills bacteria and tenderizes the meat. Use one-quarter cup of vinegar for a two to three-pound roast, marinate overnight, then cook without draining or rinsing the meat.

269). Cook tender ribs/stew meat
For extra tenderness with boiling ribs or stew meat add a tablespoon of white vinegar.

<u>BROWN CIDER VINEGAR: COOKING I</u>

<u>COOKING TIPS</u>

<u>Cooking with vinegar</u> fits in well for those who want their food to reflect a natural healthy lifestyle. Vinegar in any kitchen is a versatile, tasty and healthy ingredient that has endless culinary uses.

270). <u>A Major ingredient</u> that adds zest to condiments such as Tomato ketchup and mayonnaise.

271). <u>Mayonnaise Retrieval</u>
Get the Last remaining contents of mayonnaise or salad dressing out of the jar by vinegar and shaking.

272). <u>Homemade sour cream</u>
Blend together 1 cup cottage cheese with 1/4 cup skimmed milk and 1 tablespoon of vinegar.

273). <u>Storing Herbs in vinegar</u>
Drying the herbs. Add warmed vinegar to make sure all leaves are immersed. Use tarragon and white wine vinegar.

274). <u>Wine Substitute</u>
When a recipe calls for wine, you can substitute vinegar, diluting 1-part vinegar to 3 parts water

275). <u>White sauce</u>
Give some extra zest to your white sauce by adding ½ teaspoon of white distilled vinegar.

276). <u>Make buttermilk</u>
Add a tbsp of vinegar to a cup of milk & let it stand 5 min to thicken

277). <u>Buttermilk Substitute</u>
A great buttermilk substitute can be made by simply adding 1 tablespoon of apple cider vinegar to 1 cup of fresh or canned evaporated milk, let the mixture stand for 10 minutes or until thick.

278) British French Fries
Add drops malt while distilled vinegar on fries and/or fish in as an addition or sans ketchup- that's how the British eat them.

279). Prolong the life of potatoes
Prevent discoloration of peeled potatoes by adding a few drops of vinegar to the water. Refrigerate!

280). Eradicate cooking smells
Get rid of cooking smells by letting a small pot of vinegar and water simmer on the stove.

281). Fried Foods
Make fish less greasy by adding a tablespoon of vinegar to the deep fryer or skillet before adding the oil.

282). Pimento Peppers
An opened jar of pimento peppers can be kept for weeks if they are covered with vinegar and refrigerated.

283). Rising Bread
To help bread rise, add 1 tablespoon vinegar for every 2 ½ cups flour, when adding other liquids, reducing those liquids accordingly. Gluten elasticity.

284). Homemade Bread
Add a sheen to the crust of homemade bread by brushing the top bread with vinegar several minutes before done, then return to the oven for baking.

285). Mashed Potatoes
After the last hot milk has been added to mashed potatoes, add a teaspoon of vinegar & beat a little.

FRESHEN YOUR FISH

286). Canned fish & shrimp freshly caught taste by soaking in a mixture of sherry and 2 tbsp of vinegar.

287. Soak fish in vinegar and water before cooking for a tender, sweeter taste an excellent flavor. This will keep your hands from getting that fishy smell.

288). Freshly caught fish with vinegar before cleaning and scaling it. Rubbing with vinegar 5 minutes before scaling trick.

SCALING FISH
289). When cooking, add a tablespoon of apple cider or white wine vinegar to fried or boiled fish.

BURNT FISH

290). Poor bachelor's cooks, I have blackened fish without a recipe. Vinegar in a towel, twirled about the head will stop the smoke detectors.

291). Freshens the air and captures the smoke smell before the whole house is caught.

292). Cleaning Fish
Before scaling fish, rub with vinegar to make scaling easier & hands from getting that fishy smell.

293). White Fish
Add 2 tablespoons of vinegar to 1-quart water, soak for 20 minutes to keep fish white and fish fresh.

294).<u>Lemon substitute</u>

Replace a lemon by substituting 1/4 teaspoon of vinegar for 1 teaspoon of lemon juice

295). <u>Preserve peppers</u>

Put freshly picked peppers in a sterilized jar and finish filling with boiling vinegar

296). <u>Firmer gelatin</u>

Firm up gelatin by with a tsp of vinegar per box.

297). <u>Improve the flavor of cooked fruit</u>

Add a spoonful of vinegar when cooking fruit.

298). <u>Great pie crust</u>

Add 1 tablespoon vinegar to your pastry recipe.

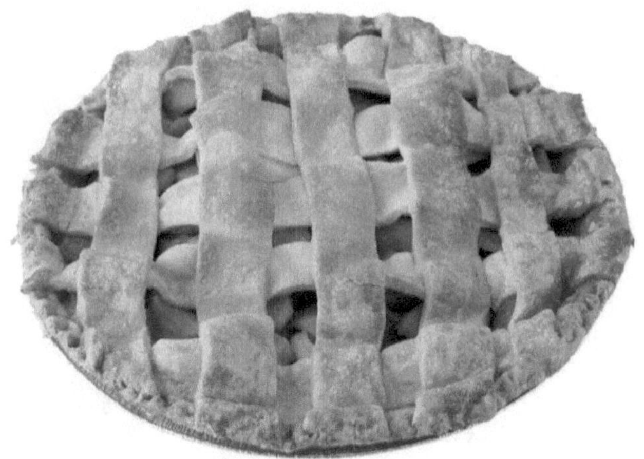

Homemade Pasta is not only fun and easy recipe to make in your own kitchen,

But nothing compares to the taste and texture of fresh homemade pasta.

Stir the pasta As the pasta starts to cook,

Stir it well with the tongs so the noodles

Don't stick to each other (or the pot).

299). <u>Prepare fluffier rice</u>

Prepare fluffier rice by adding a teaspoon of vinegar to the water when it boils or add apple cider vinegar or rice vinegar.

300). <u>Foolproof Pasta</u>

When making pasta, add 1 tablespoon of vinegar to the cooking water to avoid adding salt.

301). <u>Less Starchy Pasta</u>

Add a dash of white distilled vinegar to the water to prevent stickiness.

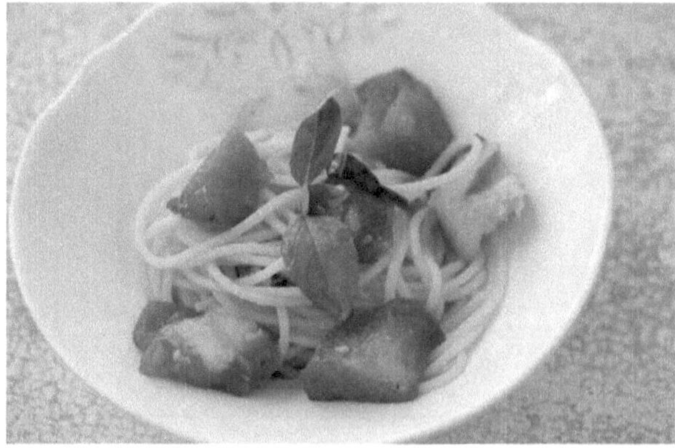

302). Salads
Make creamy vinaigrette by adding some plain or whipped cream to a mixture of 1-part white distilled vinegar to 3 parts oil.

303). Avoid lingering cabbage smells
Avoid cabbage smells by adding vinegar to the cooking water

304. Make wine vinegar
Make wine vinegar by mixing 2 tablespoons of vinegar with 1 teaspoon of dry red wine

305). Delicious Potato Salad
To make a perfect potato salad dressing, combine 1 cup mayonnaise, 2 tablespoons white distilled vinegar, 1 tablespoon sugar, ¼ cup mustard, ¼ cup sweet pickles, ½ teaspoon salt.

306). Better Deserts
You can reduce excess sweetness of pies by adding a teaspoon of vinegar to the recipe.

307). Better Pie Crusts
Pie meringue are fluffier by adding 1 teaspoon of vinegar for every 3 egg whites.

308). Foolproof Pie Crusts
Pie crust can be made flakier by adding 1 tablespoon of vinegar to the recipe.

309). Moistness for Cakes
Add moistness to any chocolate cake with vinegar

310). Cake Frosting Magic
To keep frosting from sugaring by adding a teaspoon of vinegar. keep white frosting shiny,

<u>**VEGETABLE COOKING I**</u>

311). <u>Clean vegetables</u>

Remove bugs from vegetables by washing them in vinegar and salt. The bugs should float.

312). <u>Flavor Enhancer</u>

Thyme vinegar provides an aromatic flavor

313). <u>Fungal growth</u>

Thyme vinegar deters fungal growth

314). <u>Eliminate grease tastes</u>

Add vinegar to your deep fryer stops greasy taste

315). <u>Fluffy meringue</u>

For fluffy meringue, beat 3 egg whites with a teaspoon of vinegar

316). <u>Olives preserver</u>

Olives/pimentos will keep indefinitely with vinegar and refrigerated

317). <u>Soup Gourmet</u>
Perk up any can of soup with a teaspoon of red or white wine vinegar.

318). <u>Soup Enhancer</u>

Splash into soup as a tranquilizer for frazzled nerves.

319). <u>**MY HOMEMADE VEGETABLE SOUP**</u>

<u>(FOOLPROOF): MEDIUM CROCK POT</u>

¼ Cup Apple Cider Vinegar

1 Can tomato soup (Italian seasonings)

1 Small Can Creamed corn

1 Can Cream of Chicken Soup

1 large diced fresh potato

1 cup frozen okra

1 tbsp. diced Garlic

1 cup frozen diced onion

¼ Cup cooking Wine

¼ Cup Butter (if desired)

½ Cup Water

<u>MY HOMEMADE VEGETABLE SOUP + APPLE CIDER VINEGAR</u>

There have been a number of claims made about the

Ability of apple cider vinegar

To cure illness such as the common cold or

Reduce the duration of a sore throat.

320). <u>Clean coffee makers</u>
Vinegar can help to dissolve mineral deposits that collect in automatic drip coffee makers. Fill the reservoir with vinegar and run it through a brewing cycle. Rinse thoroughly with water when the cycle is finished

321). <u>Improve your dishwasher</u>
Clean the dishwasher by running a cup of vinegar through the whole cycle once a month to reduce soap   build up on the inner mechanisms and on glassware.

322). <u>Deodorize the kitchen drain</u>
Pour a cup down the drain once a week. Let stand 30 minutes and then flush with cold water

323). <u>Eliminate onion smells</u>
Eliminate onion smells by rubbing vinegar on your fingers before and after slicing.

324). <u>Disinfect chopping boards</u>
Clean and disinfect wood cutting boards by wiping with vinegar solution.

325). <u>Keep jars free from bacteria</u>
Clean and disinfect wood cutting boards by wiping with vinegar.

326). <u>Cleaner dishes</u>
Cut grease and smells on dishes by adding a tablespoon of vinegar to hot soapy water

327). <u>Clean a teapot</u>
Clean a teapot by boiling a mixture of water and vinegar in it. Wipe away the grime

328). <u>Remove lime from kettles</u>
To remove lime coating on your tea kettle, add vinegar to the water and let stand overnight

329). <u>Eliminate garbage disposal smells</u>
Clean and deodorize the garbage disposal by making vinegar ice cubes & feed them down the disposal; grind and run cold water.

330). <u>Keep a garbage disposal clean and fresh.</u>
Mix one cup of Vinegar in water to fill an ice cube tray, freeze the mixture, grind the cubes through the disposal, and flush with water.

331). <u>Clean and deodorize jars</u>
Rinse mayonnaise and mustard jars with vinegar when empty

EVERYDAY KITCHEN CLEANING USES II

332). <u>Freshen a lunchbox</u>
Freshen a lunchbox by soaking a piece of bread in vinegar and let it sit in the lunchbox .

333).<u>Lunchbox Alternative</u>
Soak a paper napkin in Heinz Vinegar and leave it inside the closed lunch box overnight.

334). <u>Clean fridge</u>
Clean the refrigerator by washing with a solution of equal parts water and vinegar; wash the shelves and walls with that 50/50 solution.

335). <u>Clean Top of Refrigerator</u>
Cut the grime on the top of the refrigerator with a half and half solution of water and while distilled vinegar.

336). <u>Clean pots and pans</u>
Get stains out of pots by filling the pots with a solution of 3 tablespoons of vinegar to a pint of water. Boil until stain loosens and can be washed away.

337). <u>Clean & Shine (½ Hour Pot Cleaner)</u>
Clean food-stained pots and pans by filling the pots and pans with vinegar and let stand for thirty minutes; rinse in hot, soapy water.

338). <u>Clean the microwave</u>
Clean the microwave by boiling a solution of 1/4 cup of vinegar and 1 cup of water in the microwave. This should loosen any splattered-on food and remove lingering smells.

339). <u>Prevent soapy film on glassware</u>
Prevent soapy film on glassware by placing a cup of vinegar on the bottom rack of your dishwasher, run for five minutes and then run through the full cycle

340). <u>Clean aluminum utensils</u>
The minerals found in foods and water will often leave a dark stain on aluminum utensils. This stain can be easily removed by boiling a solution of 1 tablespoon of distilled vinegar per cup of water.

341). <u>Remove stains within bottles</u>
Unsightly film in small-bottles & containers can be cleaned by pouring vinegar into the bottle and shaking.

342). <u>Freshen your bread box</u>
After cleaning the bread box, keep it smelling sweet by wiping it down with a cloth moistened in vinegar

343). <u>Keeping a clean oven</u>
Grease build-up in an oven can be prevented by wiping with a cleaning rag that has been moistened in distilled vinegar and water

344). <u>Clean kitchen worktops</u>
A cloth soaked with vinegar for sanitizing kitchen counters, stoves and bathroom surfaces. This is just as effective as the anti-bacterial products and does not promote resistant; this is also a cheaper way.

345). <u>Stains on hard-to-clean utensils</u>
Stains on hard-to-clean glass, aluminum, or porcelain utensils may be loosened by boiling in a solution of one-part vinegar to eight parts water. The utensils should then be washed in hot soapy water

Vinegar-Laundry Basics: Vinegar is a veritable powerhouse when it comes to pre-treating stains,

Softening water, and boosting regular laundry detergents. When cleaning fabrics, distilled white

Vinegar or ACV is preferred, (**Please note:** Do not use on any dry-clean-only fabrics.)

346). <u>Prevent lint from clinging to clothes</u>
Add one cup of vinegar to each wash load. Reduce lint buildup and keep pet hair from clinging to clothing   by adding vinegar to last rinse.

347). <u>Moldy Wet Laundry</u>
Forgot that you left the wet laundry in the machine and it now smells moldy? Pour a few cups of white distilled vinegar in the machine and wash the clothes in hot water; run a normal cycle with detergent

348). <u>New clothes</u>
Some new clothes may be treated with a chemical that can be irritating to sensitive skin. Soak new clothing in 1 gallon of water with 1/2 cup vinegar.

349).<u>Keep bright colors from running</u>
Soak clothes in full strength vinegar for 10 minutes before washing.

350). <u>Brighten fabric colors</u>
Add 1/2 cup vinegar to the rinse cycle.

351). <u>Static cling</u>
A good way to control static cling is to add 1/2 cup of vinegar to the last rinse cycle of your wash.

352. <u>Take grease off suede</u>
Dip a toothbrush in vinegar and gently brush over the grease spot

353). <u>Remove tough stains from clothes</u>
Gently rub on fruit, jam, mustard, coffee or tea stains and then wash clothes normally.

354). <u>Brighten dingy dishcloths</u>
Get stained white socks and dingy dishcloths white again. Add 1 cup while distilled vinegar to a large pot of water, bring it to a boil and drop in the articles. Let soak overnight.

355).   <u>Remove mustard Stain</u>
Before washing a mustard stain, dab with white distilled vinegar.

<u>**THE PERFECT CLOTHES II**</u>

356). <u>Remove old chewing gum</u>

First soak the fabric in milk for an hour and then add a mixture of vinegar and corn flour (mixed to form a paste) to the ink stain and leave it to dry. Then wash the item in the normal manner

357). <u>Remove ink stains</u>

Get smoke smell out of clothes by adding a cup of vinegar to a bath tub of hot water and then hang the clothes above the steam.

358). <u>Remove perspiration stains from clothes</u>

Remove perspiration stains from clothes by applying 1-part vinegar to 4 parts water and then rinse

359).   <u>Remove deodorant stains from clothes</u>

Deodorant and antiperspirants stains may be removed from clothing by lightly rubbing with distilled vinegar and laundering as usual.

360). <u>Remove soap residue from Black clothes</u>

To remove residue that makes black clothes look dull use white vinegar in your final rinse.

361). <u>Rinse clothes better</u>

Clothes will rinse better if a cup of vinegar is added to the last rinse water. The acid in vinegar is too mild to harm fabrics but strong enough to dissolve the alkaline in soaps and detergents.

362). <u>Dyeing fabric</u>

When dyeing fabric, add a cup full of distilled vinegar to the last rinse to set the color.

363). <u>Yellowing Linens</u>

Use vinegar in the rinse water of tablecloths, napkins, sheets, etc. to keep them from yellowing.

364). <u>Silk</u>

Dip silks (do not soak) in a mixture of 1/2 cup mild detergent, 2 tablespoons vinegar, 2 quarts cold water. Rinse well, then roll in a heavy towel to soak up the excess moisture. Iron while damp.

365). <u>Improve your nylon hose</u>

Nylon hose will look better and last longer if 1 tbsp of vinegar is added to the rinse water.

366). <u>Improve creases in clothes</u>

To obtain a sharper crease in your fabrics, dampen them with a cloth wrung out from a solution of 1/3 distilled vinegar and 2/3 water. Place a brown paper bag over the crease and iron

367). <u>Eliminate iron shine</u>

To prevent clothes from becoming shiny when pressed with an iron, spray a cloth with a mixture of one- part vinegar to two parts water and place the cloth over the garment before pressing.

368). <u>Remove excess suds from clothes</u>

Excess laundry suds that develop during hand laundry by splashing a little vinegar.

369). <u>Freshen up your sweaters</u>
To deodorize a wool sweater, wash the sweater and then rinse it in equal parts vinegar and water

370). <u>Remove tailoring marks</u>

After a hem or seam is removed, there are often unsightly holes left in the fabric. These holes can be removed by placing a cloth, moistened with distilled vinegar, under the fabric and ironing

371). <u>Fabric Softener Replacement</u>

Use the same amount of vinegar as you would fabric softener plus twice the amount of water (so 2 parts water, 1-part vinegar) and put it in the softener dispenser. Clothes with reduce static

372). <u>Clothes softener</u>

Add 1/2 cup of vinegar to the last rinse cycle to soften clothes.

373). <u>Delicates</u>

If you're washing delicate items by hand, follow the garment's instructions, and add 1 or 2 tablespoons   of vinegar to the last rinse to help remove soap residue.

APPLE CIDERVINEGAR (ACV)

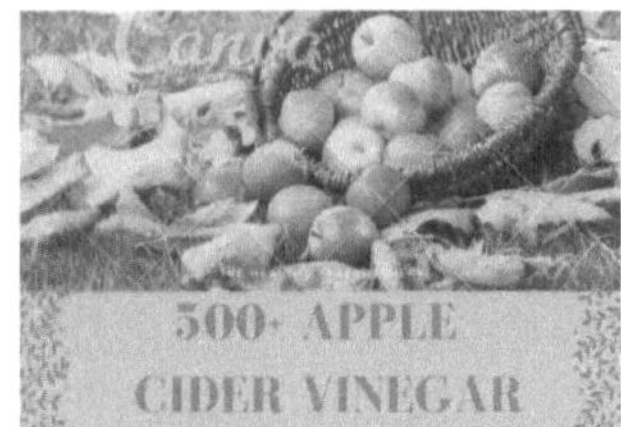

Apple cider vinegar is so great for

Curing acne because it

Returns the acidity to our skin and

Restores that acid mantle.

It also kills bacteria,

Removes excess dirt,

Oil and makeup and

Dissolves dead skin cells.

If you suffer from acne and want to make the

Apple Cider Vinegar toner that cured acne.

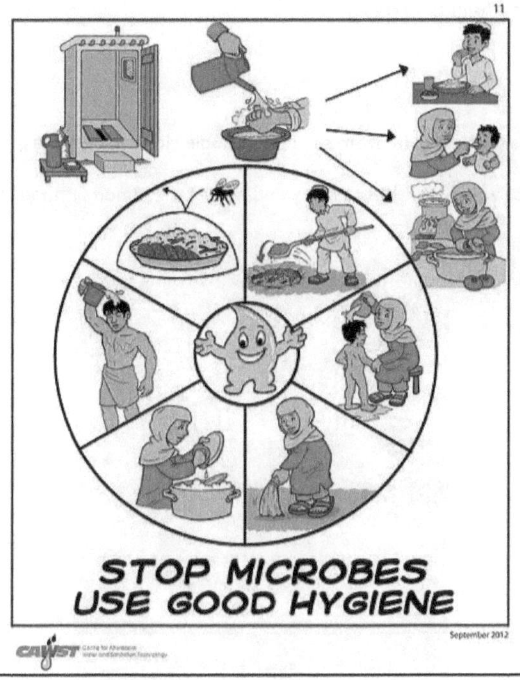

374). Aftershave Itch

Commercial aftershaves cause rashes and itching, use undiluted white vinegar as an aftershave lotion.

375). Eliminate Acne

Wash the affected area first and then dab it with a solution of 2 tablespoons of white vinegar and a cup of water. The water should be boiled first and left to cool. Repeat several times a day

377). Remove cold sores quicker

To help dry and out the cold sore, dab the affected area with gauze soaked in diluted white vinegar.

378). <u>Weight loss</u>

Vinegar naturally helps to remove fat from the body – apple cider vinegar is especially good for this.

Drink some in a glass of water a few times a day and add a little lemon or honey for a nicer flavor.

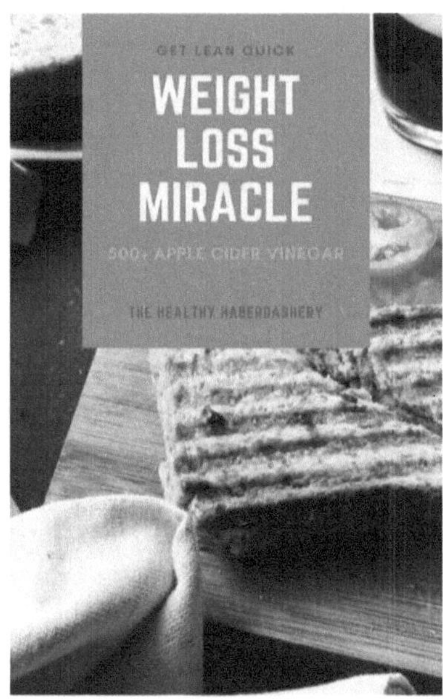

379). <u>Clean dentures</u>

Clean dentures Soak dentures overnight in Heinz White Vinegar, then brush away tartar with a toothbrush

380). <u>Shrink varicose veins</u>

Pour undiluted vinegar both onto your hands and onto the affected area and then massage the affected area thoroughly with your hands

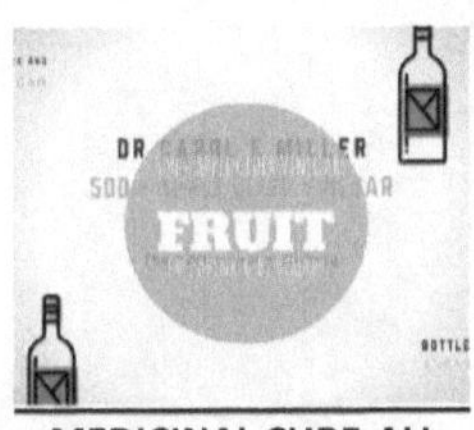

MEDICINAL CURE-ALL

PERSONAL TOXIN REMOVAL & ACV I

381). <u>Reduce Mucous</u>
Upon rising drink, the apple cider vinegar cocktail.

383). <u>Nasal Wash</u>
Mix 50/50 apple cider vinegar + water in a glass & sniff right up the nostrils until passages are clear.

384). <u>Nose Bleeds</u>
Soak cotton or gauze in apple cider vinegar and pack nostrils. Lie down 10 minutes & press nostrils.

385). <u>Eye Wash</u>
For Cataracts, mix 50/50 solution of apple cider vinegar and water, apply to the ear with an ear dropper purchased from the drug store.

386). <u>Nail Polish Extender</u>
Make nail polish last longer. Wipe fingernails with cotton balls dipped in while distilled vinegar before putting on nail polish.

387). <u>Great Body Detergent</u>
Cleans out the arteries to help reduce cholesterol.

388). <u>Increases Potassium</u>

Apple cider vinegar will increase potassium levels.

389). <u>Cures the Overweight</u>
Apple cider Vinegar acts as a fat flusher when taken 3 times a day

390). <u>Combats the Underweight</u>
Apple Cider vinegar and liquid iodine will normalize the body weight

391). <u>Relieves Headaches</u>
Headaches are alarms that tell the person that deep-down destruction.

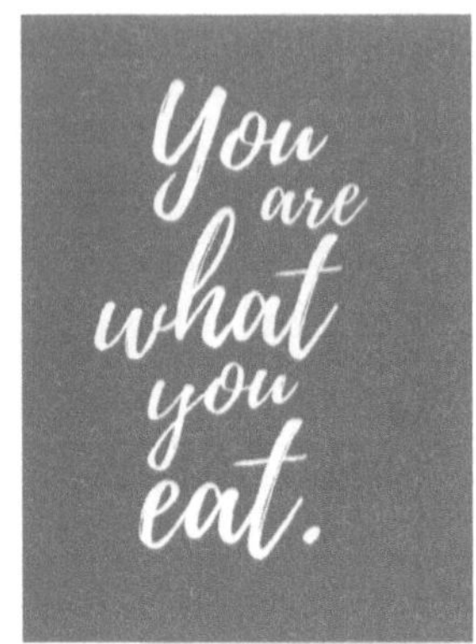

PERSONAL TOXIN REMOVAL & ACV II

392). <u>Relieves genitals</u>
Use cotton ball to apply apple cider vinegar and water (50/50 solution) and apply directly to genitals.

393). <u>Open Facial Pores</u>
To open pores & loosen dirt on face, use 3 tsp. to 1 quart for steaming pores & squeeze blackheads.

394). <u>Chicken Pox</u>
Use cotton ball to apply apple cider vinegar & water (50/50 solution), apply directly to cotton ball.

395). <u>Psoriasis</u>
Equal parts water and apple cider vinegar spray. (50/50 solution in sprayer bottle). .

396). **Poison Oak**
Equal parts water and apple cider vinegar spray. (50/50 solution in sprayer bottle).

397). <u>Dry Skin</u>
Make a paste of apple cider vinegar & add cornstarch to thicken.

398). <u>Oily Skin</u>
Drink apple cider vinegar to balance the Ph level for an ongoing facial treatment.

399. Hives
Drink apple cider vinegar to balance the Ph level for an ongoing facial treatment.
400).   Windburn, chapped skin
Mix apple cider vinegar and olive, apply with cotton ball.

401). Middle Ear Infections
Mix 50/50 solution of apple cider vinegar and water, apply to the ear with a cotton ball.

402). Summer's Ear
Mix 50/50 solution of apple cider vinegar and water, apply with an ear dropper from the drug store.

403). Hemorrhoids
Mix 50/50 solution of apple cider vinegar and water, apply to the rectum with a cotton ball. If possible, make a paste to be used as a suppository.

404). Rectal Itching
Mix 50/50 solution of apple cider vinegar and water, apply with a cotton ball.

405). Diaper Rash
Mix 1 tsp apple cider vinegar and wet swab to apply 3 times a day.

406).Fungus Infection
Mix 50/50 solution of apple cider vinegar and water, apply to the area with a cotton ball.

407).   Jock Itch
Mix 50/50 solution of apple cider vinegar and water, apply to the area with a cotton ball.

408).   Athletes Foot
Mix 50/50 solution of apple cider vinegar and water for a lukewarm soak.

409).   Mouth Thrush
Gargle every 3 hours with 1 tsp. apple cider vinegar and ½ glass of warm water.

410).   Eczema
Mix 50/50 solution of apple cider vinegar and water, apply to the affected area twice a day.

411).   Bladder problems
Mix 1/3 tsp. of apple cider vinegar in 1 glass cranberry juice.

412).   Shrink Prostrate
Mix 50/50 solution of apple cider vinegar and water, apply to the affected area.

413). <u>Sits Bath:</u>

ADD 1 CUP APPLE CIDER VINEGAR TO SOOTHE ACHING BODY.

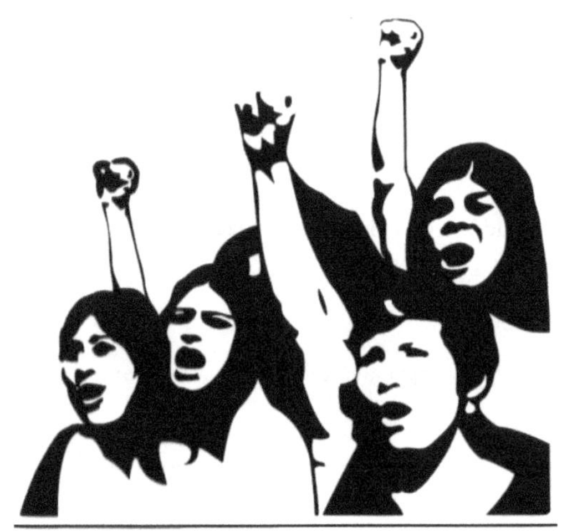

414). <u>HOT FLASHES</u>

DRINK THE APPLE CIDER VINEGAR COCKTAIL AT LEAST 3 TIMES PER DAY.

415). <u>PMS</u>

DRINK THE APPLE CIDER VINEGAR COCKTAIL AT LEAST 3 TIMES PER DAY.

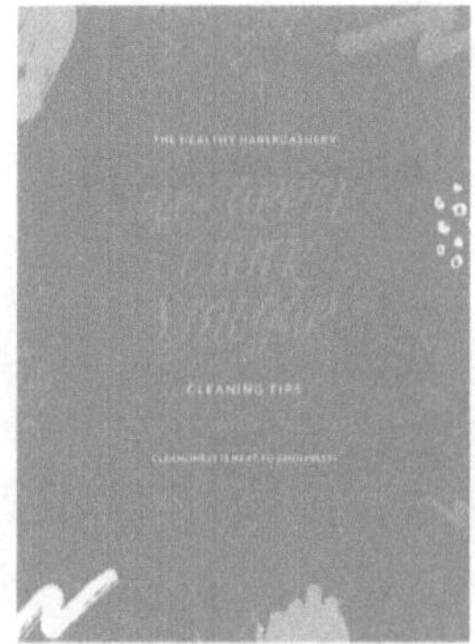

CHILDREN TOXIN REMOVAL I

416. Clear away crayon stains

You can get these stains off by rubbing them with a recycled toothbrush soaked in undiluted vinegar before washing them.

417). Clear away pen ink

First wet the spot with some white vinegar, then rub 2 parts vinegar to 3 parts cornstarch. Let the paste thoroughly dry before washing.

418). Clear away bloodstains

Before a bloodstain sets in, treat it by pouring full strength white vinegar on the spot. Soak 5-10 min.

419). Remove rings from collars and cuffs

Scrub your shirt collars & cuffs with a paste of 2 parts white vinegar & 3 parts baking soda. Let the paste soak for ½ hour before washing.

Scrub your clothing with a paste of 2 parts white vinegar and 3 parts baking soda. Let the paste soak for half an hour before washing

KIDS COLORING EGGS

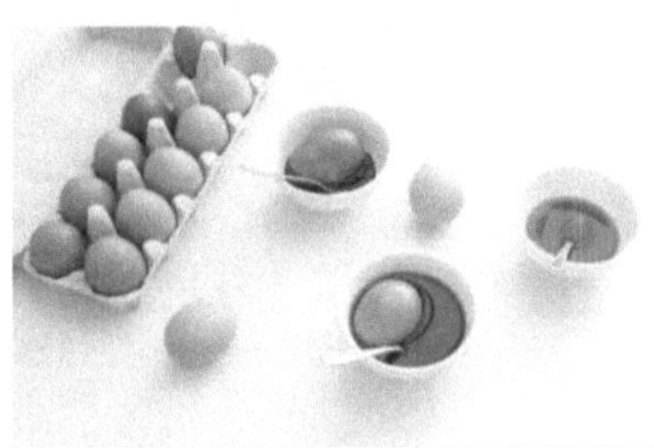

421). **COLORING EGGS**

Mix 1 tsp of vinegar with each ½ cup of hot water, then add food coloring. (Check egg-coloring food dye directions). Vinegar keeps the food dyes bright and prevents streaky, uneven colors.

422). Making Naked Eggs

Place eggs in a container so the eggs are not touching. Cover the eggs with vinegar. Spoon to scoop the eggs out. Be careful since the eggshell has been dissolving. Carefully dump out the vinegar. Put the eggs back in the container & cover them with fresh vinegar. Leave the eggs in the refrigerator for another 24 hours!

423). <u>BUILDING A VOLCANO</u>

First, make the "cone" of the volcano: Mix 6 cups flour, 2 cups salt, 4 tablespoons cooking oil and 2 cups of water. The resulting mixture should be smooth and firm (more water may be added if needed).Stand a soda bottle in a baking pan and mold the dough around it into a volcano shape. Do not cover the hole or drop dough into it. Fill the bottle most of the way full of warm water, add red food color Add 6 drops of detergent to the booth contents. Add 2 tablespoons baking soda to the liquid. Slowly pour vinegar into the bottle. Watch out – eruption time.!

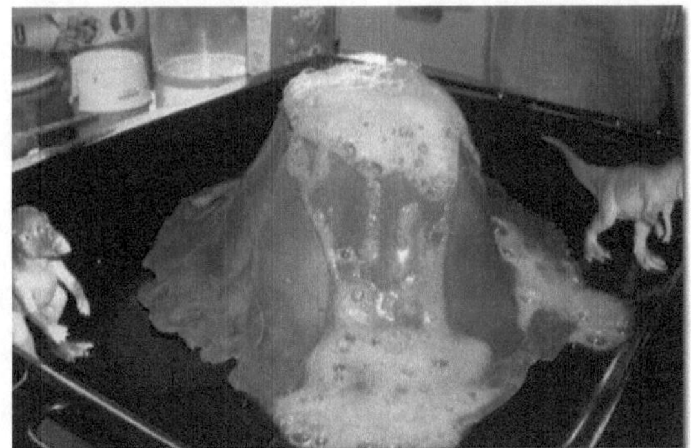

424). A LITTLE VINEGAR ON THE TONGUE OF A SASSY PRESCHOOLER WORKS WELL AS SOAP!

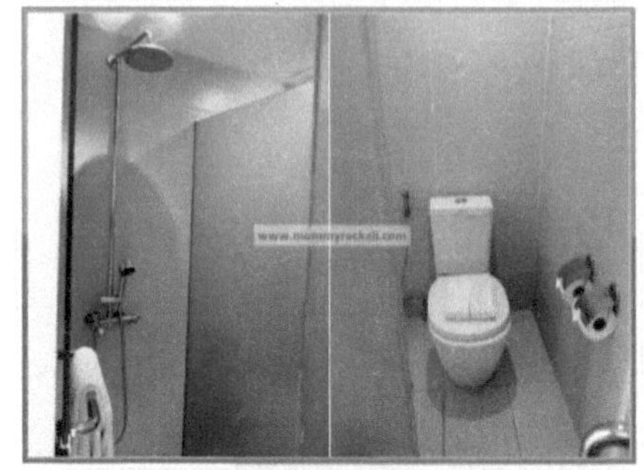

425). <u>Remove soap stains</u>

Soap & stain build up can be removed from chrome & fixtures with 1 tsp of salt & 2 tbsp vinegar.

426). <u>Kill bathroom germs</u>

Kill germs on fixtures by using 1-part vinegar to 1part water in a spray bottle. Spray the bathroom fixtures & floor, then wipe clean

427). <u>Clean a slimy sponge or loofah</u>
Soak it in a strong solution of vinegar and water for a day, then rinse times in cold water, dry in the sun.

428). <u>Remove bathroom mildew</u>

Clean soap scum, mildew, and grime from bathtub, tile, and shower curtains. Simply wipe the surface with Vinegar and rinse with water

429). <u>Remove stubborn toilet stains</u>

Stubborn stains can be removed from the toilet by spraying them with vinegar & brushing vigorously. The bowl may be deodorized by adding 3 cups of vinegar. Allow it to remain for ½ hour & then flush.

<u>EVERYDAY BATHROOM CLEANING II</u>

430). <u>Unclog a shower head</u>

Unclog a shower head by unscrewing it, remove the rubber washer, place the head in a pot filled with

equal parts Vinegar and water, bring to a boil and then simmer for five minutes.

432). <u>Metal Corrosion</u>

Corrosion may be removed from showerheads or faucets by soaking them in diluted distilled vinegar

overnight. This may be easily accomplished by saturating a terry cloth towel in vinegar and wrapping

it around the showerhead or faucet

433). <u>Remove bath tub film</u>
Bath tub film can be removed by wiping with vinegar and then with soda. Rinse clean with water

434). <u>Clean bathroom surfaces</u>
A cloth soaked with vinegar for sanitizing kitchen counters, stoves and bathroom surfaces. This is just

as effective as the anti-bacterial products and does not promote resistant strains like the commercial

products can.

435). <u>Water Rings</u>

Combine vinegar & olive oil, use solution on a soft cloth to wipe away stains.

436). <u>Glass showers</u>

Shower doors can be cleansed with alum & vinegar – 1 tsp alum + ¼ cup vinegar.

HEALTHY GARDENING TIPS I

437). <u>Grow beautiful Azaleas</u>
Occasionally water plants with a mixture of 2 tablespoons vinegar to one-quart water.

438). <u>Plants</u>
A squirt of vinegar may help invigorate a plant and make it more resistant to disease and pests. Mix 1-ounce vinegar with 1-gallon compost tea .

439). <u>Kill grass on paths and driveways</u>
Pour full strength on unwanted grass. Kill grass or weeds by pouring hot vinegar on it. This might take a couple of times to work completely.

440). <u>Clay Pot Cleaning</u>
Remove white salt build-up on old clay pots by soaking them in full strength vinegar

441). <u>Kill weeds</u>
Spray full strength on growth until plants have starved. Boil 1-quart water, then add 2 tablespoons salt and 5 tablespoons vinegar. Hot water, pour directly onto weeds between the cracks on sidewalks

442). <u>Deter ants</u>: Use spray bottle, ants hate the smell of vinegar.

443). <u>Cats</u> can wreak havoc on your garden by using it as a litter box. Soak wads of newspaper with vinegar and scatter them in areas where the cats have been. The vinegar smell should discourage repeat visits.

444). <u>Cockroaches;</u>
A squirt of pure vinegar from a spray bottle may stop a cockroach to be captured and disposed.

445) <u>Slugs</u>
Slugs like to feed on gardens at night or on cloudy, damp days. To combat them, fill a spray bottle with   half vinegar & half water. Search out slugs at night.

446).   <u>Increase soil acidity</u>
In hard water areas, add a cup of vinegar to a gallon of tap water for watering acid loving plants like rhododendrons, gardenias, or azaleas.

447). <u>Seedlings</u>
If seedlings begin to mold clean them with 1-part vinegar to 9 parts water and transfer them to a new container. Spritz seeds while awaiting germination.

<u>HEALTHY GARDENING TIPS II</u>

448). <u>Freshen cut flowers</u>

Add 2 tablespoons of vinegar and 1 teaspoon of sugar for each quart of water

449). <u>Roses</u>

Mix 3 tablespoons natural apple cider vinegar in 1-gallon water. Fill garden with sprayer of the mixture and spray the roses daily to control black spot or other fungal diseases.

450). <u>Prolong the life of flowers in a vase</u>

Add two tablespoons of vinegar plus three tablespoons of sugar per quart of warm water.

451). <u>Water line in flower vase</u>

Get rid of water line in a flower vase by filling it with a solution of half water and half white distilled vinegar by soaking a paper towel in white distilled vinegar and stuffing it into the vase so contact with the water line.

452). <u>Neutralize garden lime</u>

Rinse your hands liberally with vinegar after working with garden lime to avoid rough and flaking skin.

Clean pots before repotting and rinse with vinegar to remove excess lime

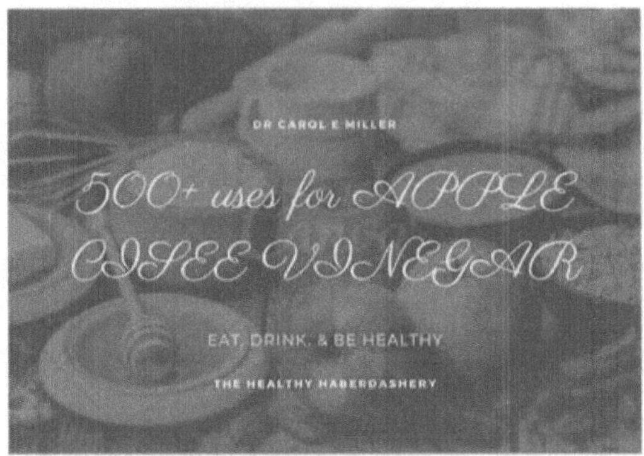

Apple cider is, essentially, an unfiltered apple juice

that tends to have a stronger flavor, which is why

we can't get enough of apple cider cocktails.

It is a popular ingredient in mixed drinks,

particularly for warm cocktails

That are delicious on cold days.

453). <u>Remove fish tank residue</u>
Eliminate that ugly deposit in the gold fish tank by rubbing it with a cloth dipped in vinegar rinsing.

454). <u>Remove animal urine stains from carpet</u>
Blot up urine with a soft cloth, flush several times with lukewarm water, then apply a mixture of equal parts vinegar and cool water. Blot up, rinse, dry

455). <u>Remove skunk odor from a dog</u>
Rub fur with full strength vinegar and then rinse

456). <u>Keep cats away</u>
Sprinkle vinegar on an area to discourage cats from walking, sleeping or scratching on it

457).<u>Stop Cats from fighting</u>
Stop cats from fighting each other with a spritz of white distilled vinegar and water solution.

458). <u>Stop dogs from scratching ears</u>
Clean the inside of the ears with a soft cloth dipped in diluted vinegar

459). <u>Keep away fleas and mange</u>
Add a little vinegar to your pet's drinking water

460). <u>Keep chickens from pecking each other</u>
Stop cats from fighting each other with a spritz of white distilled vinegar and water solution.

461). <u>Clean pets cages</u>
Use a mixture of 50% White Vinegar and 50% Water in a spray bottle to clean the pets cage.
It disinfects and deodorizes it and is much cheaper than the commercial products

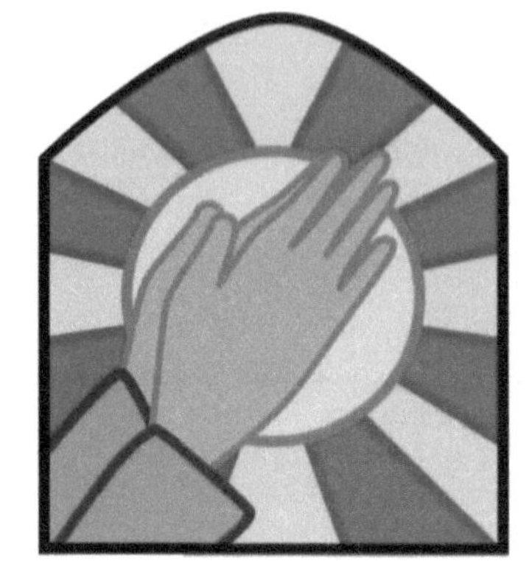

462). Hand Stain Remover

Stain remover: If your hands are stained from chopping berries, dab some straight apple cider vinegar on the stains and they'll disappear like magic. Tired, swollen hands or feet: Rub on ACV.

463). Overnight facial

Get rid of blemishes and make your skin more youthful by patting apple cider vinegar on your face before bed. You'll have softer skin in the morning!

464). Sunburn bath

When singed by the sun, find soothing relief by adding a cupful of ACV, soaking for 10 minutes.

465. **<u>DANDRUFF FIGHTER ACV</u>**

Mix 1-part apple cider vinegar to

3 parts warm water

to balance scalp pH and control dandruff.

You can also apply undiluted

ACV to the scalp.

Allow it to penetrate, then

shampoo with a mild shampoo.

<u>APPLE CIDER VINEGAR</u>

Apple cider vinegar for dandruff is the best thing you can use to get rid of dandruff quickly.

These convenient and easy-to-use natural remedies of dandruff

Will give you relief from the scaly scalp and

Leave you with healthy looking hair.

Dandruff is estimated to affect up to 50% of people.

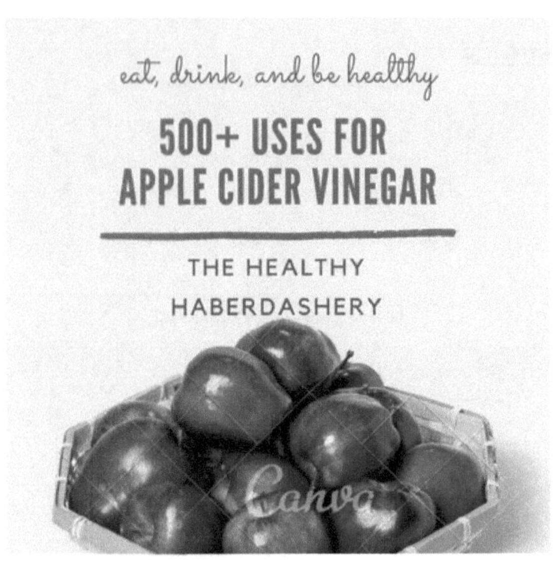

<u>APPLE CIDER VINEGAR FOR DANDRUFF</u>

Apple cider vinegar also has anti-inflammatory properties that help soothe an aggravated scalp of

irritation and inflammation. More often than not, an oily scalp is the reason behind scalp flaking.

Apple cider vinegar prevents this by helping balance oil production in the scalp.

Apple cider vinegar is effective in getting rid of dandruff because the enzymes present in it are so

powerful that they are capable of killing both bacteria & fungal infections. The main reason that is

believed to be the cause of dandruff is the excessive production of. yeast on the scalp.

ACV contains antimicrobial, antiviral, and anti-fungal materials that fights yeast directly.

466.Pet Care with Apple Cider Vinegar

As a pet care product, apple cider vinegar (ACV) is hard to beat for its versatility, availability and cost. Use the unfiltered, organic ACV that has not been pasteurized for best results. ACV should not be fed however, to a pet who is sensitive or allergic to **yeast** or one who has a chronic yeast infection. In these cases it is believed that the vinegar can feed or exacerbate the problem .Here are some of the more common benefits you can derive by using apple cider vinegar as a natural product for both cats and dogs.

APPLE CIDER VINEGAR IS DAILY HEALTHINESS.

As an ear care product.

As pet care to fight fleas and ticks.

It can be relief for skin problems.

Use it for skunk odor removal.

As an ingredient to reduce weight.

To improve dog fertility.

To remove cat urine spray.

467. PET CARE - DAILY HEALTH TONIC
The minerals, enzymes and acids in unpasteurized apple cider vinegar can supplement your pet's existing diet. It can be added either directly to the dog's food or drinking water.

468). PH; a good source of easily absorbable potassium, apple cider vinegar aids digestion, inhibits the growth of unfriendly bacteria: helps maintain the proper acid/alkaline balance of the digestive tract.

469). Show dogs I don't want to shave I use 50% Apple Cider Vinegar, 50 % water mixed in a spray bottle, several times daily.

470). Dog Toy
Soak a chicken bone is a glass of vinegar for 3 days. It will bend like rubber for your dog to play with.

471). Dog Gas
Rub apple cider vinegar on a dog's stomach – where the hair is sparest and within ½ hour, the dog should be a more socially acceptable companion.

472). **<u>HOLISTIC VETS RECOMMEND A DAILY DOSAGE</u>:**

1 tsp (5 ml) for cats and small dogs
(up to 14 lb.)

2 tsp (10 ml) for medium dogs
(15 to 34 lb.)

1 tbsp (15 ml) for large dogs
(35 to 84 lb.)

NOTE: DO NOT FEED ACV TO DOGS THAT HAVE IRRITATION OF THE INTESTINAL TRACT LINING.

473). <u>Pet Care - Ear Care Product</u>
Unfortunately, a large percentage of dog and cat visits to the veterinarian are for ear problems, but the good news is, you can help reduce these visits by cleaning your pet's ears on a regular weekly basis. An inexpensive way to do this is to dip a soft cotton ball into a solution of equal parts apple cider vinegar and water and use it to swab the inside of his or her ear. For an infected ear, use 5 ml of the 50:50 vinegar water solution per 20 lbs. (9 kg) of body weight, applying the solution with a syringe obtained from your local pharmacy. Gently rub in the solution then wipe the inside of the ear with a soft cotton ball. This should be done daily for 5 days. The vinegar helps to control the growth of unfriendly bacteria and other microorganisms that are a common cause of ear infections, and as a result, this will help keep your pets from scratching.

474). <u>Pet Care - Fleas and Ticks</u>
Rather than use commercial sprays, powders, pills or collars that use very toxic chemicals to kill fleas and ticks, many people prefer to take a more natural holistic approach. Add to an 8-ounce bottle of your favorite pet shampoo, 10 drops of tea tree oil and one tablespoon (15 ml) of aloe Vera and shake well. Shampoo your pet as you would normally then wait for 6-10 minutes. Rinse with apple cider vinegar diluted in water. (1 tablespoon ACV to 1 pint of water)

475). <u>Minor flea infestations</u>
Another recommendation involves washing your pet with a gentle shampoo, followed by a thorough rinse then spraying on apple cider vinegar diluted with an equal amount of warm water. Allow the pet to drip or shake dry. The fleas will drown in the soapy shampoo water and the vinegar rinse will acidify your pet's skin making it very unattractive to other fleas and ticks.

476). <u>Pet Care - Relief for skin problems</u>
For dry itchy skin, hot spots, or skin infections you can bathe your pet in warm water then rinse him or her with a solution of 1-part ACV to 3 parts water. This vinegar rinse will also leave their coats soft and shiny.

477). Pet Care - Skunk Odor Removal

Bathing your dog or cat in tomato juice is the most widely used method to remove the sharp smell of skunk from any pet that has had an unfortunate run in with a skunk. If you are caught without a supply of tomato juice, don't fret, vinegar can be used as well. Many authorities recommend you sponge **undiluted vinegar** into his coat and skin. Be careful not to get the solution in your pet's eyes, allow it to dry and then follow with a mild pet shampoo and warm water rinse.

478). Pet Care - Slimming down Ingredient

For those dogs and cats that need to lose weight, Robert S. Goldstein V.M.D., and Susan J. Goldstein have written an excellent article on how to help your pet lose those unwanted pounds and become happier and healthier along the way. They include a slimming supplement that you can make at home that is made from kelp, lecithin, vitamin B6 and organic apple cider vinegar.

479). Pet Care - Improved Dog Fertility

Dr. D. C. Jarvis, in his popular book Folk Medicine, recounts the story of a dentist friend of his who was having problems breeding boxer dogs. He had five females in his kennels and only one litter had been born in the last year. Dr. Jarvis, thinking that this was due to a lack of potassium and other minerals, suggested that the ration of each dog be reinforced daily with one tablespoon of apple cider vinegar. During the following year all five female boxers produced litters and the puppies were born strong and vigorous.

480). Pet Care - Remove Cat Urine

If your cat (or dog for that matter) urinates on your favorite carpet or couch, apply or spray white vinegar onto the soiled area as soon as possible.

Allow it to soak for 10 minutes to absorb the odor and loosen the stain then blot it up with paper towels. Repeat if necessary. Always test the vinegar on a small section of carpet or fabric first to make sure it does not fade the existing colors.

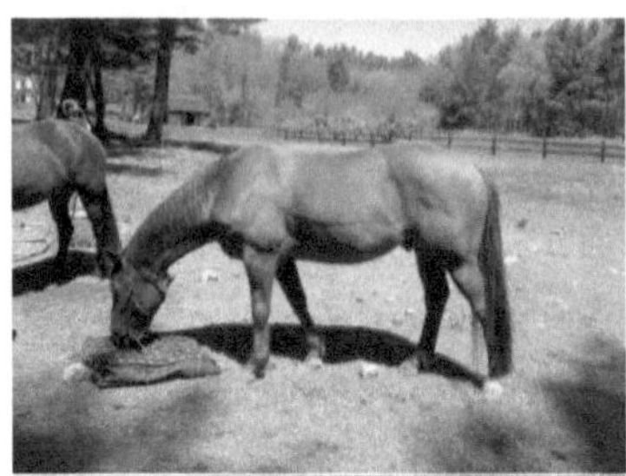

481).<u>HORSE CARE USING APPLE CIDER VINEGAR I</u>

How is apple cider vinegar used for horse care? The nutritional bounty found in unpasteurized apple cider vinegar (ACV) is not only good for people, it's beneficial for horses as well.

HERE ARE WAYS THAT ACV IS USED TO HELP HORSES:

It's a nutritional supplement for feed and water.

It helps prevent intestinal stones called enteritis.

It's a natural horse fly spray.

It's a mild cure for skin conditions

It's an excellent horse hoof care product

482). Horse Care – Water and Feed Supplement

Dr Jarvis, the Vermont country doctor on the use of apple cider vinegar in his book *Folk Medicine*, found that a horse would chew the wood of his stall because the wood contained potassium.

483.   Experimenting with calves

He found that they would not chew the wood of their pens if ACV was added to their drinking water, since apple cider vinegar is an excellent source of easily absorbable **potassium** trace minerals.

484). <u>Horses, recommended dosage</u> rates vary from 1 cup (250 ml) of ACV for every 50 gallons (190 liters) of drinking water all the way up to 1 cup (250ml) for every 6 gallons (23 liters). For a horse that will not drink the water in a new location, a commonly used tip is to add apple cider vinegar.

For a healthy horse, use 1/4 cup (60 ml) of unpasteurized ACV on his feed grain per day. Dilute the vinegar 50/50 with water.

485. Feed for Foals

Because of its potassium and associated trace mineral content, this feed supplement is for mares coming up to foaling and it is also beneficial for **older horses** with digestive difficulties or arthritis.

HORSE CARE USING APPLE CIDER VINEGAR II

486). Horse Care – Intestinal Stones
Intestinal stones called *enteroliths*, can develop in susceptible horses which can cause blockages that require expensive surgery. Since the ingestion of vinegar increases the **intestinal acidity** in horses, it helps prevent these stones from forming according to veterinary researchers at the University of California at Davis. The number of horses developing enteroliths has increased over the last 10 years especially in certain geographical areas such as the southwestern part of the United States, particularly California. As well, certain breeds such as Arabians and Moroccans seem to be more prone to enteroliths than others.

487).Horse Care – A Natural Fly spray

Another benefit of feeding your horse apple cider vinegar is to make the horse less attractive to flies and insects. Specialists believe that horses sweat the vinegar out so that it becomes a natural horse fly spray. Insect bites not only cause your horse itchy discomfort, they can be areas where skin bacterial and fungal infections can occur. As well, types of hives are commonly caused by insect stings or bites.

They can cause other health risks by spreading such diseases as West Nile virus, encephalomyelitis viruses and equine infectious anemia. Never use a commercial fly repellant containing DEET on horses (or other animals) since it can be absorbed or ingested by them causing toxic side effects.

488). **INSECTICIDES ON HORSES**

For those who prefer not to use insecticides for horse care, especially on foals less than 12 weeks old, try feeding your horse ACV and make up your own vinegar based natural horse fly spray that you can rub or spray onto your horse's coat:
2 cups (500 ml) Apple Cider Vinegar
1 cup (250 ml) Water
1 cup (250 ml) Avon Skin so Soft (bath oil)
2 tsp. (10 ml) Eucalyptus oil (or citronella oil).
Mix all ingredients & store in a handy spray bottle.

489).Pesky flies on horses

You can take care of all those pesky flies that hang around enclosed areas like barns & trailers, by making homemade vinegar fly traps:

3 cups (750 ml) Water

1/4 cup (60 ml) Apple Cider Vinegar

1/4 cup (60 grams) Sugar

Dissolve the sugar in the vinegar solution then place in a large jar and punch holes in the lid. The flies will get in but won't be able to fly out.

<u>**HORSE CARE USING APPLE CIDER VINEGAR III**</u>

490). <u>Identify the type of insect on horses</u>

Or the species of fly
bothering your horse
because they all have their
own preferred breeding spots
& feeding times,
then use the appropriate
horse care tips.

491). <u>Horse Care for Natural Fly Protection</u>

Eliminate insect **breeding sites** by covering manure piles and disposing of them often.
Remove daily from stalls and pens all manure, and waist hay then spread thinly or and compost.
Eliminate standing water that can collect as cans, old tires, discarded bedding wet material.
Stable horses at sunrise and sunset which are peak feeding times for black flies, no-see-ums, mosquitoes. Install overhead stall fans to interfere with the insect's flight. Place fine mesh screens windows. (60 Squares/in2) Use fly masks, bonnets, body sheets that does not allow the flies to reach the skin.

492). <u>Horse Care – Mild Cure for Skin Conditions</u>

Full strength apple cider vinegar can be rubbed directly into the horse's skin around a ringworm infection. Ringworm is an infection of the skin and hair by several types of **fungi** (not worms). Rub in thoroughly two or three times a day for several consecutive days. This is especially useful for ringworm infections that are too close to the eyes to use a copper wash.

493). <u>Horse Care – Horse Hoof Care</u>

Thrush and other foot fungus infections can be greatly reduced by a regular spray or soak application of apple cider vinegar to the soul and frog of your horse's feet. By making the hoof area more acidic, fungus is no longer able to grow well there. A general horse hoof soaking solution can be prepared by adding 1/4 cup (60 ml) of apple cider vinegar to one gallon (3.8 liters) of water. The vinegar application will, at the same time, speed up the healing of any other foot infections or bruises your horse might have.

494). <u>Goat Fly Repellent</u>
Feed your goat a quarter of a cup of apple cider vinegar daily, it will keep the flies away and also deter them from the goat feed.

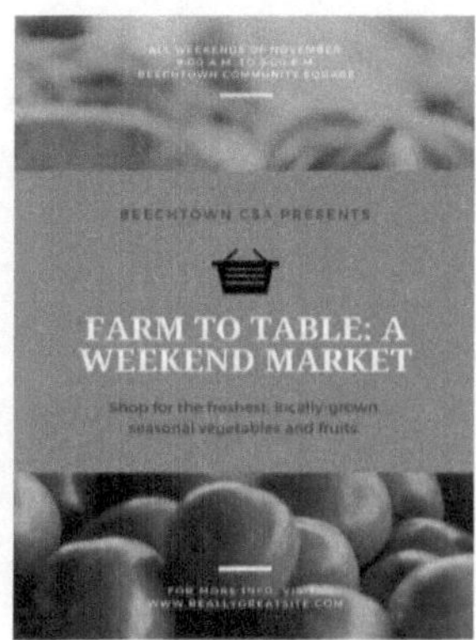

!

YOUR HUMAN HEALTH

495).<u>Allergies</u>
As an allergy to crabs, you can dip my crabmeat in vinegar, some don't get an allergic reaction.

496).<u>Backache</u>
Add two cups of vinegar to a hot tub, sit for 30 min.

497). <u>Bad Breath</u>
Simply rinse your mouth and gargle with a solution of half vinegar and half water.

498). <u>Bee Stings & Bug Bites</u>
A paste of cornstarch and vinegar applied to the itchy, irritated area relieves pain.

499). <u>Body Odor</u>
Vinegar makes a great natural deodorant. That's because its acidity kills the bacteria that causes the odor to appear in the first place. Mix equal amounts vinegar and water and dab it under your arms with a cotton ball. Let it dry completely.

500). <u>Bruises</u>
Dip a clean cloth into a bowl of chilled vinegar and apply to the bruise. Some folk healers swear that the healing process will speed up if you soak a slice of thick onion in the vinegar and then apply it directly to the bruise.

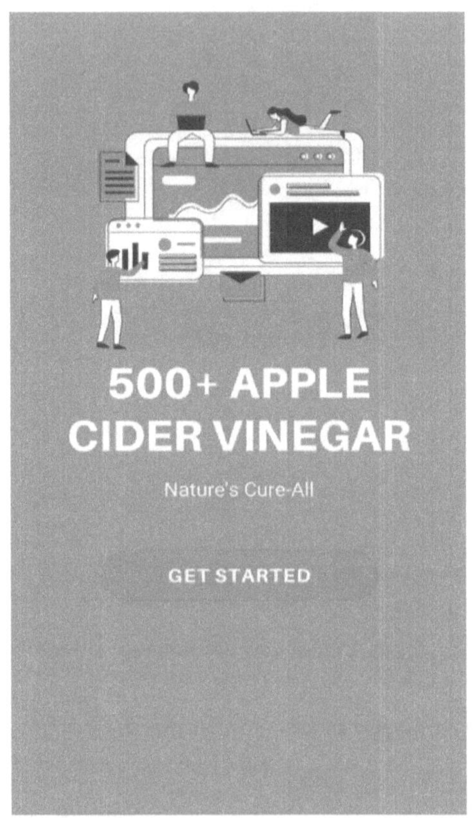

501).+ <u>ACV: COUGHING</u>
Make your own cough syrup by adding equal parts honey and vinegar to a bottle, then shake to mix. Take one tablespoon every four hours as needed.

502). <u>Cramps</u>
Apply full strength vinegar to the cramping area. The pain should subside within seconds. To prevent those painful leg cramps, drink water with 1 tbsp vinegar.

503). <u>Birth Control</u>
An ancient birth control method thought crude where women were advised to put honey, olive oil, or oil of cedar into their vaginas. Stickiness slows the movement of sperm into the uterus.

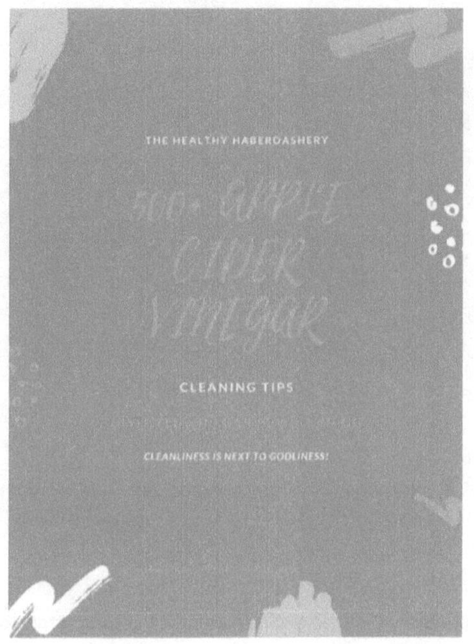

504).   <u>Homemade Tampons</u>.

Wads of soft wool soaked in lemon juice or vinegar were used as tampons, making the vagina

sufficiently acidic to kill the sperm.

505).   <u>Incontinence</u>

Bath with soap and water. Then wipe the skin with vinegar which reduces odor and prevents

bacterial growth.

506).   <u>Check calcium supplements</u>

To check the absorbability of calcium supplements, drop them into vinegar. If they dissolve quickly,

then they are of good quality.

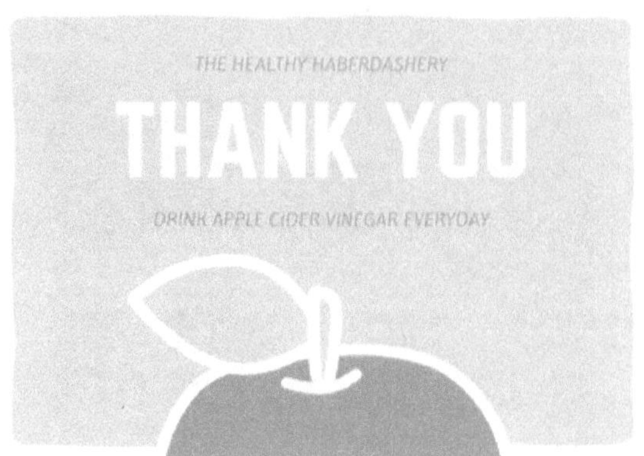

507). <u>Colds are Banished</u>!
Soak an 8-inch square of brown paper cut from a paper bag in ACV. When the paper is saturated sprinkle it with pepper and bind to the chest with cloth strips,. After 20 minutes, remove and wash .

508). <u>Liniment:</u>
Apply to sprains as a hot poultice. Wrap an afflicted area with a cloth wrung out of apple cider vinegar for 3 to 5 minutes.

509).<u>Make Saddle Soap</u>
Mix 1/8 cup linseed oil, ¼ cup beeswax, ¼ cup vinegar. Warm the beeswax, slowly in the vinegar. Add the soap and oil. Keep the mixture warm until smooth. Cool until it is solid. Rub it onto good leather, then buff toe bottom of the open edges with apple cider vinegar.

511). <u>Disinfecting socks</u>
Avoid re-infecting athletes' foot by rinsing your socks with white vinegar.

512). <u>Reinvesting Athletes Foot</u>
Avoid re-infecting feet by wiping shoes with vinegar.

513). <u>Frizz</u>
Over permed hair is untangled with a vinegar & water mix.

Numbers 6:3

[3]He shall separate himself from wine and strong drink, and shall drink no vinegar of wine, or vinegar of strong drink, neither shall he drink any liquor of grapes, nor eat moist grapes, or dried.

Ruth 2:14

[14]And Boaz said unto her, at mealtime come thou hither, and eat of the bread, and dip thy morsel in the vinegar. And she sat beside the reapers: and he reached her parched corn, and she did eat, and was sufficed, and left.

Psalms 69:21
[21]They gave me also gall for my meat; and in my thirst they gave me vinegar to drink.

Proverbs 10:26
[26]As vinegar to the teeth, and as smoke to the eyes, so is the sluggard to them that send him.

Proverbs 25:20

[20]As he that taketh away a garment in cold weather, and as vinegar upon nitre, so is he that singeth songs to a heavy heart.

<u>**VINEGAR BIBLICAL SCRIPTURES: NEW TESTAMENT**</u>

Matthew 27:34

[34]They gave him vinegar to drink mingled with gall: and when he had tasted thereof, he would not drink.

**Some think it was a way to mock Jesus, but others argue that the "vinegar" (with gall)
was the diluted wine drunk daily by the Romans, given to alleviate his pain.**

Matthew 27:48

[48]And straightway one of them ran, and took a sponge, and filled it with vinegar, and put it on a reed, and gave him to drink.

Mark 15:36

[36]And one ran and filled a sponge full of vinegar, and put it on a reed, and gave him to drink, saying, Let alone; let us see whether Elias will come to take him down.

Luke 23:36

[36]And the soldiers also mocked him, coming to him, and offering him vinegar,

John 19:29
[29]Now there was set a vessel full of vinegar: and they filled a sponge with vinegar, and put it upon hyssop, and put it to his mouth.

John 19:30

[30]When Jesus therefore had received the vinegar, he said, "It is finished": and he bowed his head and gave up the ghost!

Wine was offered to Jesus on three separate occasions.
The gospels indicate the first time He was offered wine it was mixed with gall.
The second time Christ was mocked as a king, and
The third time wine was offered to Him, it was sour wine.

References

Anon, (2020). [online] Available at: https://draxe.com/health/ph-balance/ [Accessed 17 Jan. 2020].

Healthline. (2020). *Can Apple Cider Vinegar Help You Lose Weight?*. [online] Available at: https://www.healthline.com/nutrition/apple-cider-vinegar-weight-loss#section3 [Accessed 17 Jan. 2020].

Homeopathy. [online] Available at: https://en.wikipedia.org/wiki/Homeopathy [Accessed 17 Jan. 2020].

Jcrows.com. (2020). *Herbs for Horses, Equine Herbal Formulas, Herbals for Horses*. [online] Available at: https://jcrows.com/equineformula.html [Accessed 17 Jan. 2020].

Parents. (2020). *https://www.parents.com*. [online] Available at: https://www.parents.com/recipes/scoop-on-food/7-reasons-why-apple-cider-vinegar-is-a-busy-mom-s-secret-weapon/ [Accessed 17 Jan. 2020].

Science Driven Nutrition. (2020). *Is Apple Cider Vinegar a Miracle Food? - Science Driven Nutrition*. [online] Available at: http://sciencedrivennutrition.com/apple-cider-vinegar-evidence/ [Accessed 17 Jan. 2020].